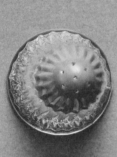
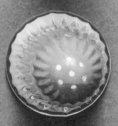
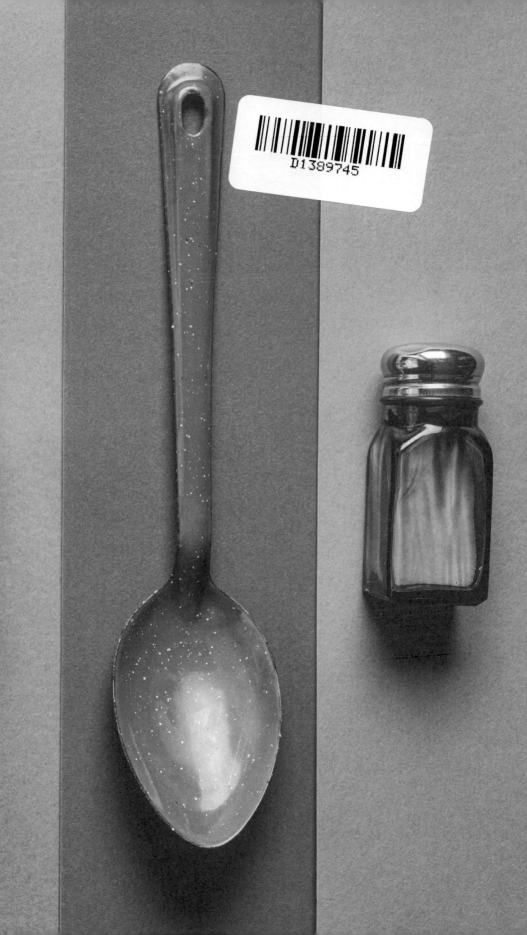

D1389745

TWOCHUBBYCUBS

TWOCHUBBYCUBS

THE COOKBOOK

100 Tried and Tested Slimming Recipes

James Anderson & Paul Anderson

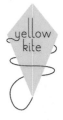

yellow kite

First published in Great Britain in 2020
by Yellow Kite, an imprint of Hodder & Stoughton
An Hachette UK company

4

Copyright © James Anderson and Paul Anderson 2020
Photography by Haarala Hamilton © Hodder & Stoughton 2020

A CIP catalogue record for this title is available from the British Library.

Hardback ISBN 978 1 529 39803 8
eBook ISBN 978 1 529 39802 1

Colour origination by Altaimage
Printed and bound in Germany by Mohn Media

Hodder & Stoughton policy is to use papers that are natural, renewable and recyclable products and made from wood grown in sustainable forests. The logging and manufacturing processes are expected to conform to the environmental regulations of the country of origin.

Yellow Kite
Hodder & Stoughton Ltd
Carmelite House
50 Victoria Embankment
London EC4Y 0DZ

www.yellowkitebooks.co.uk
www.hodder.co.uk

Notes

The information and references contained herein are for informational purposes only. They are designed to support, not replace, any ongoing medical advice given by a healthcare professional and should not be construed as the giving of medical advice nor relied on as a basis for any decision or action.

Readers should consult their doctors before altering their diet, particularly if they are on a set diet prescribed by their doctor or dietitian.

The calorie count for each recipe is an estimate only and may vary depending on the brand of ingredients used, and due to the natural biological variations in the composition of natural foods such as meat, fish, fruit and vegetables. It does not include the nutritional content of garnishes or any optional accompaniments recommended for taste/serving in the ingredients list.

Where not specified, ingredients are analysed as average or medium, not small or large. Eggs are medium and milk is semi-skimmed unless otherwise stated.

Senior Commissioning Editor: Lauren Whelan
Project Editor: Natalie Bradley
Copy-editor: Annie Lee
Nutritionist: Kerry Torrens
Internal design: Clare Skeats
Photographer: Liz and Max Haarala Hamilton
Food Stylist: Frankie Unsworth
Art Director and Prop Stylist: Jennifer Kay
Production Manager: Claudette Morris

CONTENTS

DEDICATION

This book would have been impossible were it not for the work of one woman. My mum. If she hadn't enjoyed one too many beer garden snakebites on a lusty summer night back in 1984, I wouldn't have been here at all. (I'll give you a moment while you imagine the blandness of a world without me in it …)

However, I've shown my gratitude for her snatch game many times over, through petrol station flowers and loan repayments, so while she's important, she's not the one this book is dedicated to. No, that dubious honour belongs to my nana. Long since turned to lavender-scented ash and thrown to the wind to trouble the emphysema of her mourning friends, my nana was an absolute hero of mine. If this was a fancy book, I'd tell you all about how she used to pick raspberries for my sister and me, us all laughing gaily as we burst their scarlet beads all over our cherubic faces, talking about adventures and ginger beer and the war.

But it isn't. My teenage (when I knew better) experiences with my nana involved consistently pushing Trex-laden pastry out of her hands, refusing the ton of off-brand Werther's Originals that she would proffer from her tissue-strewn pockets, and desperately trying to solve why there was always half a potato sitting in a jug of water on the worktop. She died before I ever worked that mystery out, and I can't say in all honesty that I've ever quite forgiven her.

However, she was always there for me growing up, and supported me in whatever I wanted to do: drop out of school ('You're too good for that posh place, with all those bastards in their fancy cars'); marry a bloke ('But who is the woman?'); or grow my hair so long I could sit on it ('You look as though you'd sell me pegs and read my fortune'). Nothing fazed her.

She came to our civil partnership and then proudly told everyone at the Women's Institute that I'd *finally* found a husband. I was twenty-two. Imagine the scandal that caused among people for whom modern values were a distant concept. Still, they're all dead, so who's laughing now?

But what does this sepia-tinted memory have to do with Twochubbycubs? It's because of her that it even exists. I was trying to show her how to use an iPad and I took a photo, which we turned into a comic strip using an app. Well, she thought that was tremendous, and it planted a seed that the same app could be used to make recipe cards. We gave it a go, stuck a recipe online for some awful curry loaf (a much-improved version can be found in this book) and never looked back.

Paul and I would go over and excitedly tell her that we had forty followers, a hundred, a thousand. She assumed we had joined a cult and offered to pray for us – I didn't have the heart or the patience to tell her that nothing could save my soul. When we made our first ten pounds from advertising she was absolutely cock-a-hoop, not least because she saw a future where she would get more than a box of jellied fruits for Christmas (not that she would let you buy her anything, of course).

Then, just as the blog began to really take shape, so did a bowel obstruction, and after a brief couple of days where we awkwardly stood around her hospital bed hoping she would manage a crap and be fine, she decided to nick off and see what my grandad was doing up in the clouds. (I might hold a seance and ask her if she can send me some of my old nudes from the cloud, actually. I lost them in the great Apple password leak of 2013, and damn those were the days when everything stood firm.)

We cremated her, scattered her down the West Road (accidentally, my mum dropped the urn trying to light a cigarette and a good half of her blew straight into the brushes of a roadsweeper), and all moved on. Not a week goes by without me thinking about her, and if she could see this now, and how terrifically exciting it all is, she would be proud and amazed. For about five minutes, that is. Then it would be time for *Coronation Street* at a volume that would crack concrete.

This one's for you, Dorothy B.

James

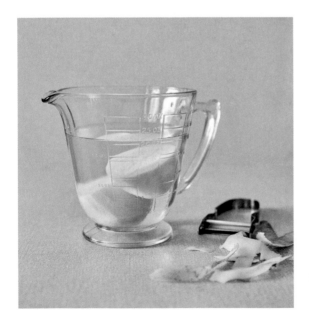

'THIS ONE'S FOR YOU,
DOROTHY B.'

James has covered the schmaltz side of things, but let's not forget why we are really here: all the hundreds and thousands of people who follow us and make it all worthwhile. All the people who wanted something different from yet another boring old recipe blog; who wanted to laugh their way through a diet rather than sob into an egg-and-sweetener cake.

We would write and post even if the only person reading our blog was the Google Indexing machine (and he never calls or writes, the bastard), but knowing that there are folks out there taking the time to scroll through our nonsense means the absolute world. We never set out to make a difference, but the sheer amount of comments, positive feedback and nudes puts a whole new spin on it. Seriously though, ladies, stop sending us fuzzy shots of your bajingos – we're not for turning.

We've had some amazing stories; our favourite is a young lad with a heart condition – hi David! – who has his mum reading our nonsense to him in his hospital bed (I presume she leaves out the dirty jokes) and who has been inspired to cook as a result. The amount of people who have said this is the first time they've ever stuck to losing weight because they realize it doesn't have to be tiresome and tasteless. Ladies and gentlemen who have stopped caring what everyone else thinks of their bodies and embraced a new lease of life, away from feeling shy and judged. It's incredible. We wake up daily to such amazing stories and comments and it just makes it all the sweeter that we love what we do.

With all that in mind, our second dedication is to everyone out there who has followed us and made what we do so enjoyable, so fun and so lucrative. You've made us smile, cry and travel the world. This is just the start – we have our eye on an American road trip, after all. James and I hope you enjoy the book and that it helps you on your slimming journey, but even if it doesn't, at least you have a nice weighty tome to kill spiders with.

Good luck, and thanks again!

Paul

KEEP IN TOUCH AND TAG US WITH YOUR TASTY CREATIONS!

- 🅕 TWOCHUBBYCUBS
- 🅞 @TWOCHUBBYCUBS
- 🅣 #TWOCHUBBYCUBS

WELCOME

We have tried to keep the style of the blog in this book – so although the photos may look fancy and the paper glossy, it's still very much us. We've been asked to tone down the swearing and perhaps ease back on the vast array of saucy jokes, but we're confident that you'll see we have managed to slip in a few here and there.

Our cookbook is different because we wanted it to be the equivalent of us coming over, fingering your curtains, looking at your tatty cutlery drawer and telling you some nonsense while you fart about making dinner. Just like our blog. All our recipes are easy, tasty and – most importantly – something you'd want to eat on a diet. They're meals to enjoy, not endure. We've included 10 classic blog recipes, these are marked with a star. If you're the type of person who can't bear all the flimflam you get with recipes where the author drones on about where they sourced their spaghetti (Lidl, since you ask), just jump straight to the recipe itself.

We aren't chefs – we need to make that clear. We've accumulated a hotchpotch of cooking skills and ideas over the years of running the blog, but you'll never find anything complicated in our recipes because frankly, Paul gets a sweat on trying to figure out how to cut a potato into wedges. To that end, you mustn't fret if you want to mix up the ingredients or try something different – it's what we do! Worst case-scenario if it all goes wrong? You get a takeaway.

Every dish featured in the book has been analysed by a nutritionist and the calorie count per serving is printed alongside the recipe. All the recipes in the book are under 500 calories per serving except for the Occasional Blow Out chapter, which is there for when you want to indulge. We're firm believers here at Chubby Towers that if you're making a lifestyle change to lose weight and keep it off, then this has to involve breaking the rules sometimes.

If you're a member of a slimming club, you'll find that the majority of our recipes are agreeable for your plans, though you will, of course, need to work these out yourself. Feel free to write notes on the recipe pages – don't feel precious about it! We haven't aimed to make these recipes as 'low' as possible because, honestly, we believe better flavour is always worth 'spending' on, but even so, old habits die hard with us and thus most of the recipes lean towards those low in calories. Funny that …

Finally, a note about the structure of the recipes – turns out it is quite tricky being the sole writer of a duo book – so if we slip into 'I' when of course we mean 'we', then we humbly apologise. As somewhat of a grammar freak, it would do my nut in too! The stories are all written by me (James) with Paul popping up for the notes.

ALL THE RECIPES IN THE BOOK ARE UNDER 500 CALORIES PER SERVING EXCEPT FOR THE OCCASIONAL BLOW OUT CHAPTER, WHICH IS THERE FOR WHEN YOU WANT TO INDULGE.

INTRODUCTION

While we're going to write as one through the book, it's difficult to do a proper introduction of each other without it sounding pretentious by writing in the third person. Please do bear with. To keep things spicy, we have typed each other's bio.

JAMES ON PAUL

Paul remains a mystery to me, even after twelve years of happy, content, at least passable, marriage. I gaze at him as he sleeps, choking away on his wattle and dribbling all over the pillows, and wonder what I did to deserve him. Because Christ, it must have been an atrocity and a half.

Each week I spend with him I find another layer I don't know about, like an endless box of Milk Tray. Which is apt, given he's 70 per cent cocoa butter and rustles when he walks. Just the other week I discovered that he had sulked so hard as a child that he didn't speak for three weeks. I've called his mother (I call her Iggy) to try to discover what set him off so I can use it in the future, but she doesn't remember. Furious. For a man for whom adventure is opening a box of After Eight mints at half seven, he doesn't half pack some surprises. They don't call him tripod because he's steady on his feet, y'know.

Paul works terrifically hard doing fancy things to help poorly people and for that, he should be applauded and held in high regard. The poor love's only reward is me huffing around his feet with the hoover and chiding him for driving a Smart car. He's tremendously loyal, eats anything I put in front of him and is wonderful around the house. I appreciate that I've just described my husband as though he was the family Labrador but actually, that's fitting, because he's also pleasant to cuddle into and keeps my feet warm at night.

Paul has undergone quite the transformation since I met him, and not simply because he's swapping his vertical height for horizontal weight. He couldn't cook – his first meal was cooked mince (no sauce, no onions, no herbs and spices – just a literal slab of grilled mince) and boiled potatoes. I thought he was joking, but he looked at me so proudly that I choked it down with a rictus grin and belly pains. Once I'd demonstrated the basics of cooking and moved him away from exclusively Chef Ding meals, he fair flourished, and it is he that produces most of the food that Twochubbycubs has become known for. So, think of my husband as you slip that fully loaded hotdog over your lips, won't you? He'll get a warm glow, and it'll make a change for his face to flush from something other than the mildest of exercise.

Nah, I'm kidding. He's all right really. For someone from the South.

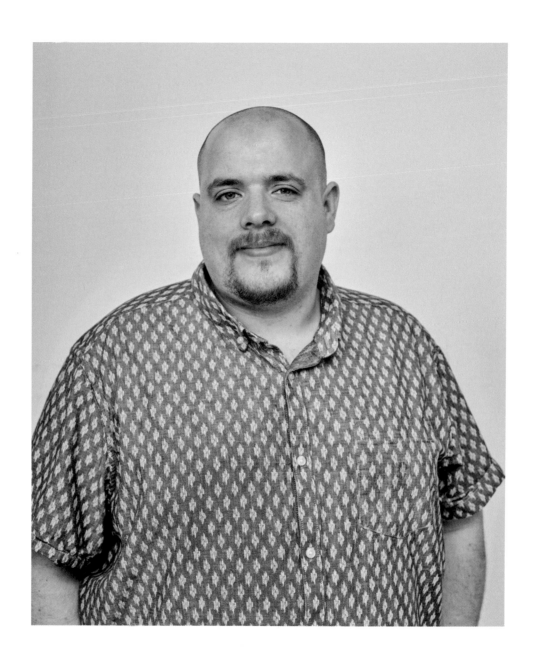

'EACH WEEK I SPEND WITH HIM I FIND
ANOTHER LAYER I DON'T KNOW ABOUT, LIKE
AN ENDLESS BOX OF MILK TRAY. WHICH IS
APT, GIVEN HE'S 70 PER CENT COCOA BUTTER
AND RUSTLES WHEN HE WALKS.'

INTRODUCTION

PAUL ON JAMES

Well, I was going to write something nice but after that I'm not sure.

As 'er indoors has already said, Twochubbycubs is a well-oiled labour of love. As one sweats away in the kitchen throwing together dinners, the other is sweating away watching YouTube clips of old *Coronation Street* episodes. Once the food has been eaten, digested and about four cigarette breaks after, James will settle down to begin writing and I think that's where the real magic starts. I'm not really quite sure how the division of labour turned out as it did – James was always the one that was the better and more adventurous cook, but over time as we developed our recipes and learned how to actually use anything other than a takeaway menu, I took over, and it's gone on from there. James tends to go down the fancier route whereas I'm more of a simple, comfort food guy, which again is the perfect metaphor for our marriage.

Now, the food is one thing but the stories that go with it, I'll admit, are my favourite part. You couldn't have Twochubbycubs without the nonsense beforehand. He's always been able to spin a good yarn – even the most boring story gets the treatment and turns into a fantastic tale of whatever, usually involving a hunky neighbour. It's worth the hassle and the tuts I get from Iggy.

As for James as a person, he's all right really. He's prone to hysterics – he once suggested burning down our house and claiming it on insurance when a spider came hurtling out from under the fridge. He's certainly a dedicated follower of fashion, if that fashion is Treasure Hunt re-runs broadcast via a dodgy satellite link. Life with him is certainly full of shock and awe – to give you an example, he surprised me with a trip to Florida when we first started dating. Always a rollercoaster, that one. He listens to far too much *Doctor Who* score than could ever be considered sensible – I can't think of a moment in our life that hasn't been punctuated by some shrill wailing and dramatic strings, although that's usually him struggling to put his boots on and crying about his thick ankles.

We've been together that long that I can't imagine a life without him. Who would rub my feet on the sofa for an hour while we watch our stories? Who would lull me into the land of nod if it wasn't him, with his cascade of belly, snoring the song of his people? Who would mock my every movement, turn of phrase? Who would get so het up at being told that 'thrice' isn't a proper word that he sulked for an entire night before sleeping in the car?

That's my James.

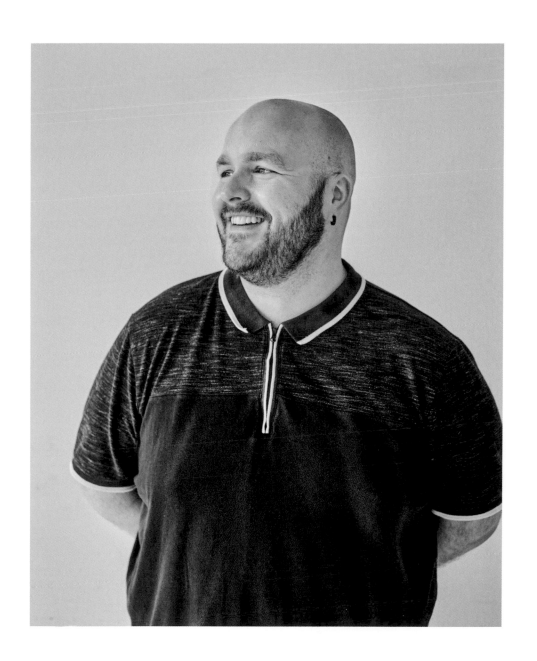

'I CAN'T THINK OF A MOMENT IN OUR LIFE
THAT HASN'T BEEN PUNCTUATED BY SOME
SHRILL WAILING AND DRAMATIC STRINGS,
ALTHOUGH THAT'S USUALLY HIM STRUGGLING
TO PUT HIS BOOTS ON AND CRYING ABOUT
HIS THICK ANKLES.'

US ON US

We're one of those awful couples that just doesn't argue and are happiest talking nonsense to each other, excluding everyone else. Smug, you might say, but we prefer lazy – you don't need to make an effort with someone you have been with for twelve years. There's no shutting the bathroom door for us or leaving the room to break wind like decent sorts.

We've seen Twochubbycubs grow from a tiny blog with eight mysterious followers (thanks Mum, Mam, Mother, Mutter, Mumsy, Chrissy69babe, retirementfund, @christIwishIhadaseconddaughter) to an unwieldy behemoth with almost half a million followers. Writing that out just seems so surreal – we remember getting excited by our first comment, for goodness sake. Now we get glorious comments all the time and it's terrific, even if we're on the verge of breakdowns from having to explain what panko is for the eight-hundredth time.

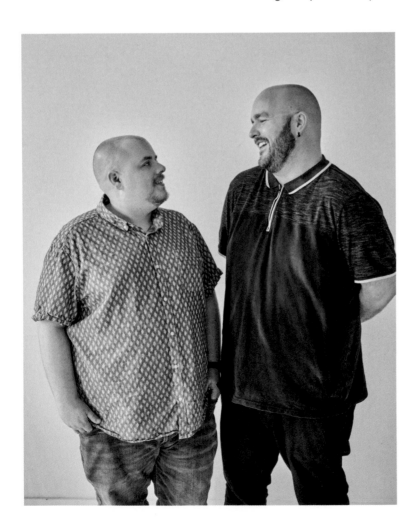

We've been stopped many times over by people in the supermarkets who shout that they love the Twochubbycubs – which, don't get us wrong, is great fun, but give us time to at least hide the pile cream, box of cucumbers and numbing spray before you bound over and cuddle us.

Ah no, we love it really.

We've also been on a very unique journey together. See, since moving in together, we steadily became more and more spherical. That's all right when you're laughing gaily at the sound of your fat slapping together during special time, more troublesome when you accidentally set the sofa on fire and you sit there hoping it'll sort itself out rather than getting up to call the fire brigade. The comfort of love leads to the discomfort of familiarity. Gosh, we'd put that on a fortune cookie but we'd only end up eating it.

Things came to a fat head in Copenhagen, of all places. Denmark, a place renowned for the super polite locals, opened our eyes to the state of our bodies. We had arranged to hire a boat to cruise up and down the river. The boat was built for four people and ran entirely on solar polar. Well. When we turned up at that jetty, all 48 stone combined of us, we saw absolute panic flash across the boat owner's face. Would solar power be enough to move us through the water? Would we even fit? How could he tell us the bad news without breaking our hearts and the wonderful Danish politeness?

He couldn't – he uttered something in broken English about maximum capacity, crossed his chest with his fingers and, after a fashion, sent us on our way. We had a merry old time pootling about the canals and waterways and actually, there must have been a nuclear explosion somewhere in the East because there was more than enough solar panel to move us about.

Disaster struck once we were finished, though. The boat owner was stood on the jetty waving his hands with significant alarm as we approached at quite the lick. Turns out we had more momentum than we had perhaps expected because we couldn't slow down in time, and crashed straight into the side. Have you seen *Speed 2*? Imagine that but with a 25-stone bearded Geordie screaming his best Sandra

'THE COMFORT OF LOVE LEADS TO THE DISCOMFORT OF FAMILIARITY. GOSH, WE'D PUT THAT ON A FORTUNE COOKIE BUT WE'D ONLY END UP EATING IT.'

> **'IF YOU FOLLOW OUR EXAMPLE: ENJOY YOUR FOOD, DON'T SCRIMP ON YOUR INGREDIENTS AND LEARN TO LOVE FOOD RATHER THAN ENDURING IT, YOU'LL BE ON YOUR WAY TO A MUCH HAPPIER WEIGHT LOSS JOURNEY.'**

Bullock impression and a 23-stone chunker trying to grab his partner by the arse-hair to stop him toppling in.

We wish the embarrassment had ended there, but as James stepped out of the boat, it tipped so violently that Paul was sent flying, and it was only after a feat of acrobatics that we would never witness again that he managed to hurl himself belly-first on to the jetty. This sight of traumatic obesity was only compounded by the fact that a hard-boiled egg, secreted from the breakfast buffet, came rolling out of Paul's trouser pocket and came to a halt at the boat owner's feet. In short, it looked like he had shat an egg out in fright.

We paid the owner handsomely for his trouble and slunk off to lick our wounds. Who could blame us – our blood was almost pure syrup at this point. But we knew we had to do something, and, surprisingly, an opportunity came up only a couple of weeks later – the chance to appear on ITV's *This Time Next Year*. The show's premise is that you pledge to do something and then film yourself over a whole year as you strive to meet your pledge, then there's a big reveal and Davina McCall starts crying and you get wheeled out in your best Next slacks and it's all exceptionally exciting.

The producers were very keen for us to take part, but rejected our initial pledge of 'we want to try a hot-dish from every country in the world' – possibly because I did a literal nudge-nudge-wink-wink when I said it. We swapped our pledge over to 'we will lose 280lb between us' – that's 20 stone, for those still using an abacus. They accepted this, recorded our initial opening bit where we sat on the sofa with Davina and made our sad faces about being so fat and chunky and delicious, and then were sent on our way, pinballing into each other as we left the studio floor. Seriously, look on YouTube, we're like two bubbles in a lava lamp.

On day one of our year, we went to Cadbury World, which should give you an indication as to how seriously we took it. It was only in month six when we received a call from the producers gently asking when we might be getting started that we realized we had to knuckle down. Our previous efforts to lose weight had resulted in losing a stone here, two stone there, the will to live entirely – the usual. It proved a tough nut to crack, which is surprising in and of itself given you're talking to two lads who can chew a chocolate orange whole and still have room for a Toblerone chaser.

It was only when we started thinking about what we were doing wrong that we decided to do something different. We had spent years making watery meals, substituting tasty ingredients for awful replacements in the vain belief that we were making lifestyle choices. We weren't.

We were kidding ourselves that the meals were worth coming home for, but instead, we were constantly snacking on unhealthy food to try to fill the void. So, with a bit of research, we decided to eat 'properly' – and the weight fell off. It was a revelation.

Which sounds over the top, but it's true. We discovered that by eating decent meals we didn't feel the need to eat rubbish on the side. Our meals were enjoyable, something to look forward to and an actual pleasure to eat. We didn't feel deprived, or that we were missing out – and the results spoke for themselves. We didn't hit our target, but we did lose 265lb between us. Davina was chuffed, we were thrilled and our local takeaway owners haven't been seen for several months.

This is where the book comes in. We were asked so many times how we lost the weight, what had we been eating, how could we assist others? We pushed back for a good few months because frankly, we needed a holiday, but then, after a brief, rewarding chat with our publishers, we agreed to set out 90 new meals from our year, together with ten classics from the blog that will help you lose weight. If you follow our example: enjoy your food, don't scrimp on your ingredients and learn to love food rather than endure it, you'll be on your way to a much happier weight-loss journey.

We hope you enjoy these meals and the chat and nonsense that goes with it. The Twochubbycubs blog has always been about having a laugh and not taking all this dieting nonsense too seriously. Life's too short to be po-faced about the food you eat, and we hope we have reflected that ethos in the book. You can come and find us online if you need more inspiration or you can pop this book straight into a charity shop window if you like – whatever works for you. But give eating well a go, and see how you get on – and tell us!

As a final note: thank you to every last one of you for believing in us. We're not ones for over-the-top sentimentality but you have no idea how amazing it feels to know that we have people trying our recipes, following our stories and loving our flimflam. We are two nondescript gay lads from Newcastle – we're not chefs, or celebrities, or anyone special – but you have made it all so worthwhile. For that we thank you, and we wish you well.

Much love

James and Paul

PS: James always comes first. But then he's always been a selfish lover.

OUR MUST-HAVES

PANS

A cast-iron casserole dish is an absolute godsend. You don't have to shell out hundreds on a fancy one, you can get them in most supermarkets. An enamelled cast-iron one is what you're after, and you'll love it like a child, trust me. For everything else, a decent set of non-stick pans is all you need.

UTENSILS

The essentials that you're going to really use are a spatula, wooden spoon, slotted spoon and a ladle. Anything else is just going to take up space in your drawers.

That said, it's worth investing in a decent knife or two. A good chef's knife and a paring knife will get you through most things. Take good care of them (don't put them in the dishwasher!) and regularly sharpen them, and they'll last you an age.

GADGETS

Here we go, the best bit. We absolutely love a gadget here at Chubby Towers and we've had most of them, so we can tell you for certain that … most of them are rubbish. HOWEVER, there are a few that are definitely worth getting:

Oil sprayer
All right, this is a given when you're on a healthy eating plan but the trick is to get the right type. Avoid anything called a 'cooking spray' – these are oils mixed with emulsifiers and propellants, which have a knack of stripping away the coating of your pans. For the best results, invest in one that you fill yourself. The 'mister' types are the best because they give a more even coating across the pan and use less. Proper cooks and chefs will probably recoil at this but I'll say it anyway – any type of oil will do. Unless you're an aficionado or using it on a salad are you really going to be able to tell the difference? If you're reading this book – the answer's probably no. And that's fine! Embrace it. Olive, rapeseed and groundnut oils are great all-rounders.

Microplane grater
Do away with fiddling and chewing on with tiny box graters and crushers and whatnot – a decent Microplane grater is all you need. They make light work of garlic and are fantastic for cheese and ginger too. Get one, you'll never look back.

Mini chopper

Too lazy to put together a whole food processor? Us too. Keep a mini chopper in the cupboard for those light bits you can't be arsed with.

Air fryer

One of the best things we've ever bought and essential if you're wanting to lose a bit of timber. For best results get the type with a stirring paddle – all the other types are inferior. They're not just for chips!

Electric pressure cooker

We were absolutely terrified of ours when we first bought it (we had it running in the garden), but don't be frightened – these aren't like that dull, dented thing your granny had screaming away on the hob. Modern ones are fantastic bits of kit that are absolutely safe and a doddle to use. You can cook so much more than a simple stew – we use ours all the time for all sorts, even yoghurt. They are worth every penny.

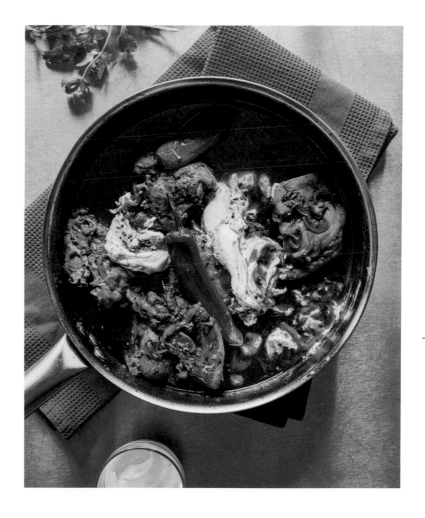

MASTER
THE BASICS

How to chop onions and garlic

A good proportion of our recipes start with sweating an onion and some garlic – it's a great foundation for any savoury dish and mastering this is your first step to becoming a great home cook. If someone had taught me how to do this properly as a kid I probably would have had enough confidence to learn how to cook properly. In fact, James had to teach me how to do it properly!

Everyone has their own technique but here's how we do it: slice your onion in half from the tip to the root, and peel off the external layers. Take each half and slice it lengthways from the top, stopping just short of cutting through the root so it stays together like a fan, then slice across. Easy. For garlic, we use a Microplane grater, which is so simple and takes seconds.

Weigh and measure

Especially important if you're trying to lose weight – don't be tempted to just guess, take the time to weigh and measure exactly. I know, I know, we can't be bothered sometimes either – but it's important.

Cook at the right temperature

Most of my early attempts at cooking resulted in burnt food because I was both impatient and not paying attention. Follow the instructions and resist the temptation to 'whack it up a bit'. If in doubt, when cooking on the hob, go lower rather than higher. Take your time!

Have everything prepped

When cooking from scratch, you can save yourself no end of hassle by having everything prepped beforehand. This stops the panic setting in of not having the next bit ready and the worry that it'll all go wrong. Read through the recipe and figure out what's needed – if anything needs a bit of prep, like slicing or chopping, we've put this in the ingredients to help you. Having little dishes of stuff ready to tip in makes you feel like a right pro and you can pretend to be on the telly and everything.

Don't be afraid to give it a go

An important one – push the boundaries. If you're a newbie and something seems a bit too difficult, give it a go anyway! Who really cares if it ends up looking like a mess?! And believe me – if I can do it, you can.

Don't be afraid to have a bit of what you fancy

This is probably the most important tip of all. If you've attended a slimming class in your life, you will be well aware of the 'substitutes' and loopholes that people try to get a taste of the things they love but that don't quite hit the mark. Don't do it! If you want a bit of cake then have a bit of cake, but have just enough to satisfy you and make sure it fits in with the rest of your eating plan. Don't try to construct a cake that looks nothing of the sort, using stuff that usually ends up in a stew, and call it a 'cake'. You'll just be eating something deeply unsatisfying, possibly not far off the real thing calorie-wise, that won't actually scratch the itch. This is something we really had to train ourselves to do but it paid off. If you want to lose weight and keep it off, you really do need to make a change for life, and being able to have 'naughty' things but in small amounts is a huge part of it.

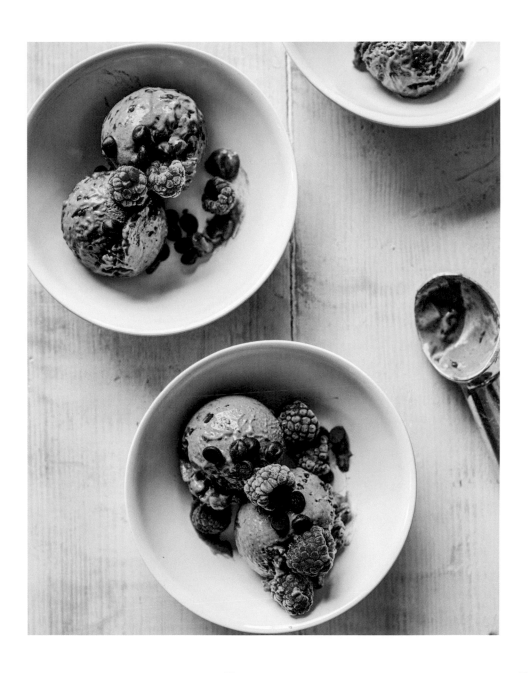

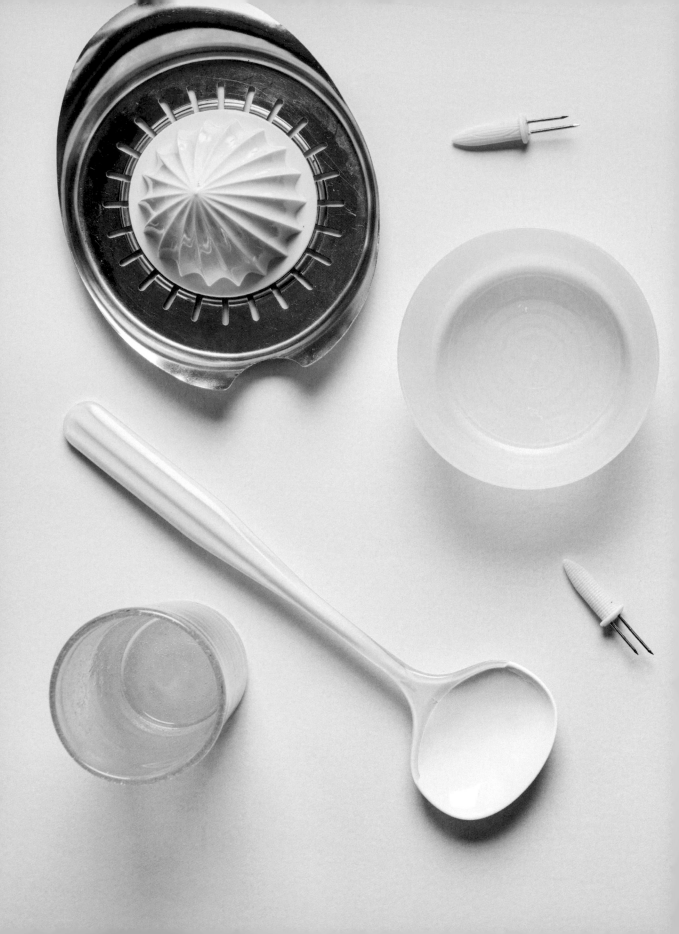

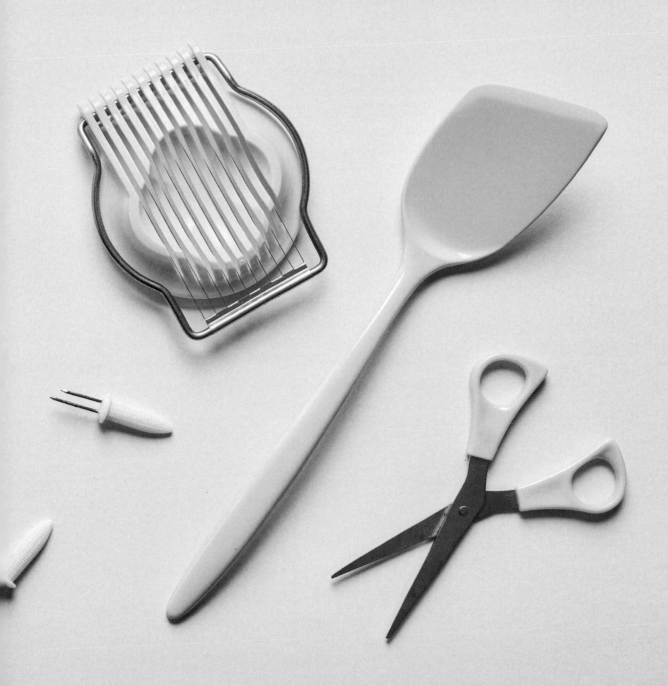

NEAPOLITAN OVERNIGHT OATS

Serves 3
348 calories

We ummed and aahed about putting an overnight oats recipe into the book – let's be frank, they're nothing more than oats, yoghurt and some tut mixed in. But see, we've been at this game for nearly five years and still people seem to struggle with the concept. You have no idea the stress caused by seeing photo after photo of people eating their 'layered' overnight oats and complaining that the oats are still dry because they haven't mixed everything together. We're not saying these people are slow on the uptake, but if you put their brain in a budgie it would fly backwards.

So, here we are. How does one jazz up overnight oats? It was only after we spent a night sobbing into a two-litre block of cheap ice cream that we hit upon the idea of Neapolitan overnight oats = chocolate, vanilla and strawberry. The freezer burn is optional, but if you want to really take the idea and run with it, you know what to do.

Now, you have three choices:
- Add the three layers to your jar, one on top of the other so you have the Neapolitan look.
- Make up each flavour variant in a separate jar and choose whichever you fancy in the morning.
- Have a bowl of Frosties and shut up.

We have found overnight oats last perfectly fine for three days in the fridge as long as they're in a good sealed jar.

150g (5½oz/1½ cups) bog-standard nowt-fancy oats (enough for 3 layers)

For the strawberry layer, place 50g (1¾oz/½ cup) oats into a screw-top jar. Finely chop 5 or 6 strawberries, then add them to the oats with a good dollop of fat-free strawberry yoghurt. Stir until it is nicely mixed and some of the juices from the strawberries run through.

For the vanilla layer, place 50g (1¾oz/½ cup) oats into a screw-top jar. Finely chop a banana, then add it to the oats with a dollop of fat-free vanilla yoghurt. Stir to combine. If you're a Waitrose shopper, you could always scrape in some vanilla seeds from the pods you invariably have on the side.

For the chocolate layer, place 50g (1¾oz/½ cup) oats into a screw-top jar. Add a handful of chocolate chips with a dollop of chocolate yoghurt (or vanilla with a touch of cocoa) and stir.

Notes from Paul
- *If you're using good fat-free yoghurt, you might find it's a little tart – a drop of honey in each layer will sort that right out more than any mountain of sweetener.*
- *We use the screw-top Kilner jars, but really, an old coffee jar will do.*
- *Add as much fruit as you like, and if you're finding it a little thick, a good splash of milk will loosen it right up.*

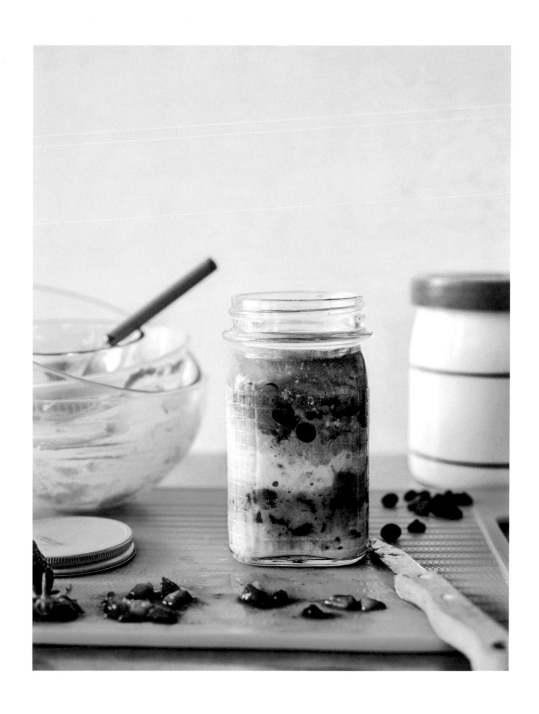

OVERNIGHT OATS ARE ALWAYS TASTY,
FILLING AND EASY TO GRAB IN THE
MORNING BUT, SEE, SO AM I, AND THE
PUBLISHERS WOULDN'T LET ME DO A
TASTEFUL NUDE CENTREFOLD.

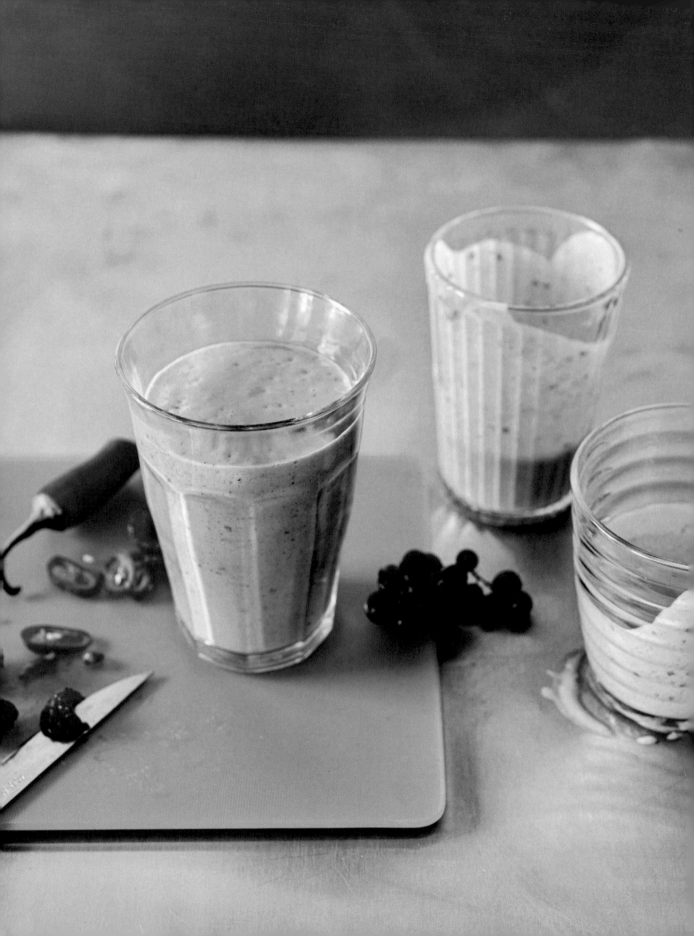

MORNING GLORY SMOOTHIES

● ● ● ● ● ●

Each smoothie serves 1

Bit of a contentious one, this, putting smoothies in a weight-loss book: we had it drummed into us over and over that smoothies are the devil's work and that by blending fruit you release all the sugar and you might as well be eating a burger made of lard for all the goodness it brings.

Now, we aren't nutritionists (I know, we were shocked to find this out too) but we're fairly confident that the same thing happens when you chew the fruit. But who knows? Either way, these smoothies are ones that we turn to when the morning is long and our willpower is weak.

We've done three smoothies below – each has an 'added extra' which shifts them up into next gear, but feel free to leave these out and enjoy a plain fruit smoothie.

Oh, and ignore the snootiness about frozen fruit – we buy it all the time and Paul's rickets have all but gone away.

145 calories

THE RING OF FIRE SMOOTHIE (opposite)

Blend together a large handful of red berries, a banana, 100g (3½oz/ ½ cup) fat-free yoghurt and some milk (depending on how thick you like it), together with a small finely diced red chilli (the extra).

171 calories

THE ORANGE-YOU-GLAD-WE-CAME SMOOTHIE (see page 30)

Blend together a handful of pineapple chunks (frozen), a banana and a peeled orange with enough milk to thin it out (or use fat-free yoghurt), and add ½ teaspoon ground turmeric and a good grinding of black pepper (the extra).

123 calories

THE LINDA BLAIR SMOOTHIE (see page 31)

Blend together a handful of spinach, a chopped apple, a few handfuls of broccoli (the extra), a handful of chopped kale and some diced frozen mango with however much milk you want, and enjoy.

Note from Paul
Nothing really to say on this one, save for the fact that it's worth buying a decent blender if you're planning on using it regularly – we started with a cheap affair (story of our life) from the supermarket and it started smoking when we had the audacity to blend anything more than mist – buy cheap, buy twice.

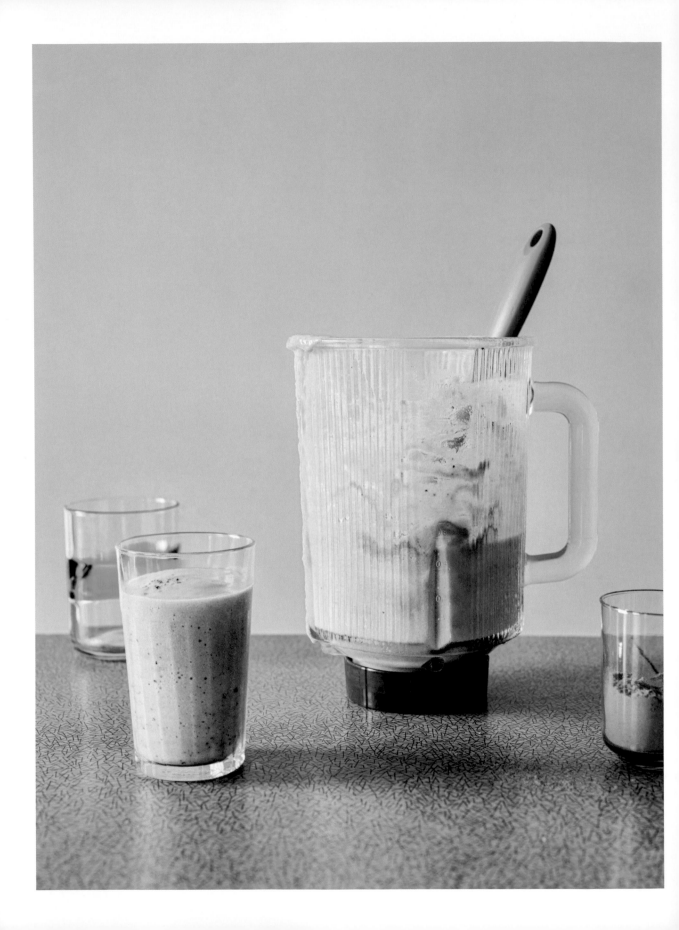

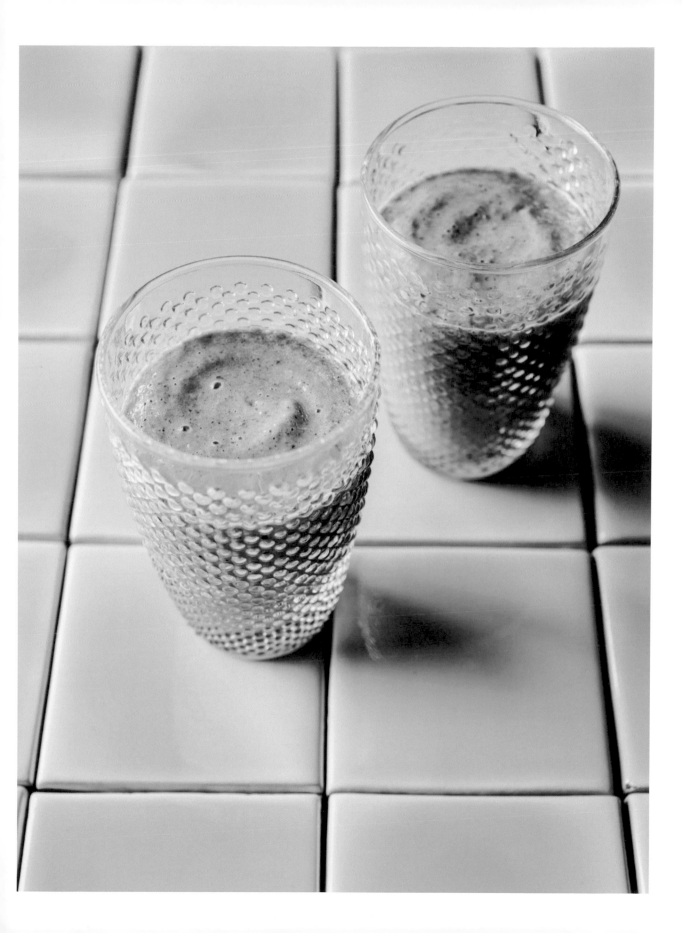

• • • • • •

DARK CHOCOLATE & ORANGE BAKED OATS

Serves 2
438 calories

1 × 298g (10½oz) tin of mandarin
   segments, drained (keeping a
   couple of spoonfuls of the
   juice to one side)
75g (2¾oz/¾ cup) porridge oats
2 small eggs
200g (7oz/1 cup) fat-free natural
   yoghurt
50g (1¾oz/⅓ cup) dark
   chocolate chips

Everyone's done overnight oats by now, and the more adventurous of you may have decided to throw them into the oven to create a baked version. The only real difference here is the addition of an egg, which binds everything together when cooked.

As usual with all of our recipes you can easily mix up the 'additions' to create new ideas – our website has all sorts of fancy ideas, including apple pie, Turkish delight and strawberry milkshake. The world is your oyster.

Preheat the oven to 200°C fan/425°F/gas mark 7 and select either 2 large ramekins or 1 large ovenproof dish.

Mix all your ingredients together, smashing up the mandarin segments as you go.

Spoon the mixture into your dishes and drizzle the reserved juice over the top. Cook in the oven for around 30 minutes, or until the top has browned nicely.

Serve to rapturous applause.

Notes from Paul
- *If you have a sweet tooth, add a tablespoon of honey to the proceedings – don't be tempted to add powdered sweetener, it makes everything taste like a chemistry set.*
- *Raspberries make an amazing replacement for the mandarin segments – there's no need to have any juice for this one, just add them whole.*
- *You know those posh desserts that come in glass ramekins – they're very handy for this.*

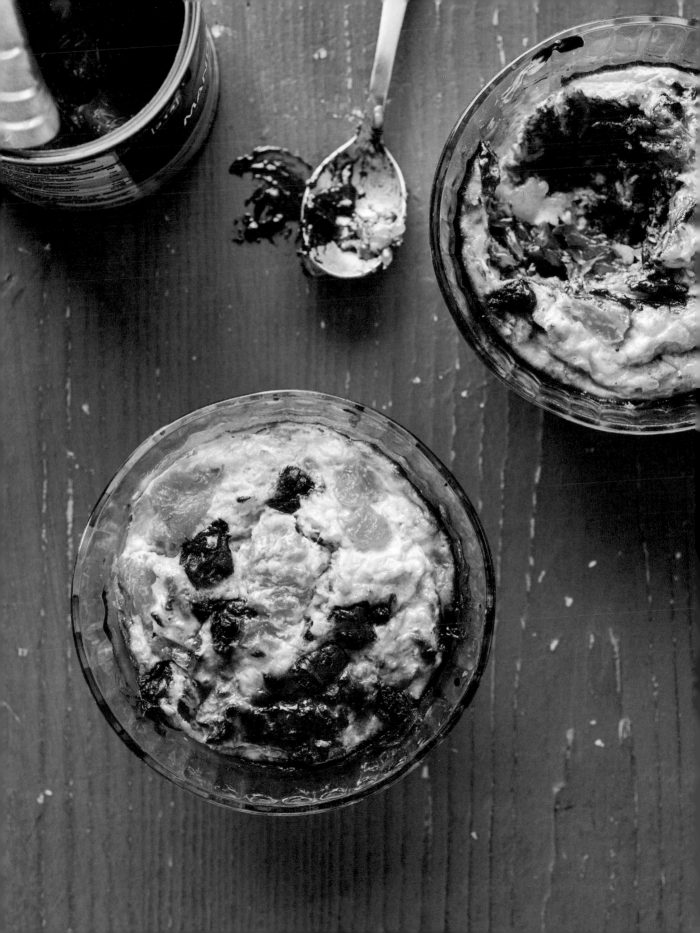

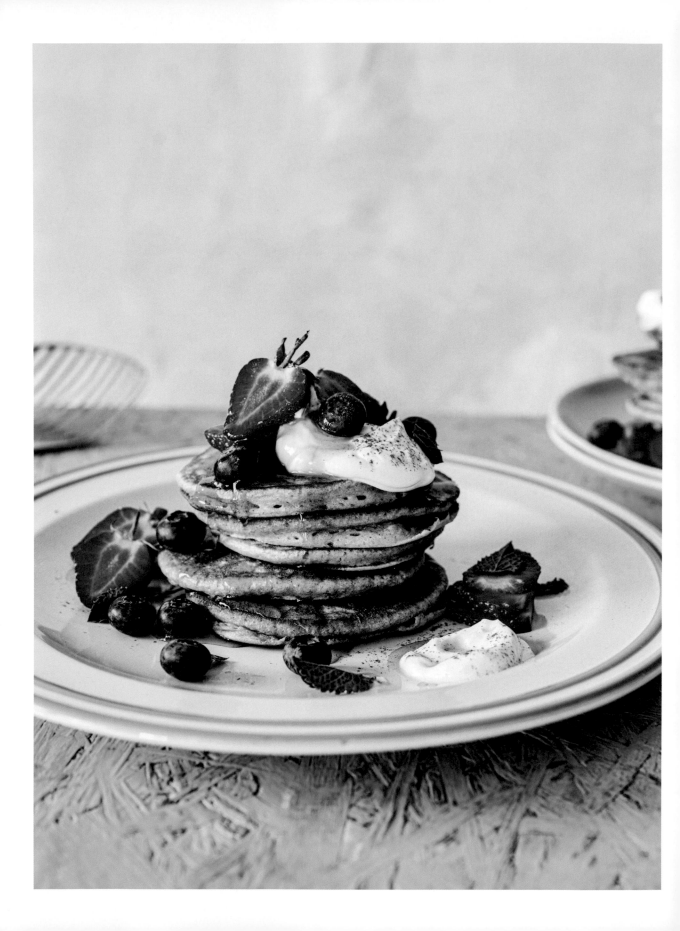

BREAKFAST PROTEIN PANCAKE STACK

Serves 4
461 calories

8 eggs
2 ripe bananas
200ml (7fl oz/¾ cup)
   unsweetened almond milk
160g (5¾oz/1½ cups) porridge
   oats
8 teaspoons baking powder
8 tablespoons fat-free Greek
   style yoghurt
160g (6oz/1½ cups) blueberries
160g (6oz/1½ cups) strawberries
2 tablespoons maple syrup
a pinch of ground cinnamon
a handful of fresh mint leaves

Pancakes have been floating around as a healthy breakfast idea for as long as I've had hair on my cheeks. Both sets.

This recipe uses almond milk but you mustn't hold that against it – you can barely taste the disappointment that comes from using non-dairy milk. Seriously, we must have tried every variation going in Paul's quest to totally ruin breakfast, though I admit to raising a suggestive eyebrow when he told me our delivery man had a load of nut milk and boy, did he need to put it somewhere. In the salad crisper, please, it's always empty.

Now listen: this recipe does make a load of pancakes, we agree, but remember that we are two workhorses when it comes to putting food away. Feel free to chip away at the ingredients if you're not quite in the mood to spend forty minutes rubbing your belly and lamenting your life choices.

Also, rather like your author, these pancakes can be topped by pretty much anything, so don't be afraid to experiment.

Put the eggs, bananas, milk, oats and baking powder into a blender and blend until smooth.

Heat a small frying pan over a medium-high heat and spray with a little oil. Pour a little of the batter into the pan to make a small pancake and cook for 2–3 minutes, then flip.

Remove from the pan and repeat the process to make a stack of 5 pancakes.

Top with 2 tablespoons of yoghurt, a quarter of the blueberries and strawberries, ½ tablespoon of maple syrup, a dusting of cinnamon and a few mint leaves.

Repeat the process to make the remaining three servings.

● ● ● ● ● ●

FIVE TOAST TOPPERS

Each topper serves 1
(on 2 pieces of rye bread)

Ah, the humble slice of toast. Too easy to drop when you're on a diet, but absolutely deserves a comeback. Don't get me wrong: if you're buttering up doorstop-sized slices of white loaf then you might be in trouble. But, swap out white bread for a decent seeded wholemeal or even – gasp – rye bread (our favourite), and top it well, you've got yourself a good breakfast.

299 calories

GOAT'S CHEESE & HONEYED BLACKBERRIES

Grab a handful of blackberries and heat them gently with a teaspoon of honey, muddling them slightly so they release some juice, then spread them over goat's cheese spread on bread.

192 calories

STEWED TOMATOES WITH A CHILLI KICK

A couple of good handfuls of tomatoes cut into chunks (a nice mix of colour always cheers the soul), 1 finely chopped red pepper and 1 very small diced red chilli pepper – simply heat everything gently in a pan with a pinch of salt and allow to bubble down. Once the tomatoes have broken down and everything is softened, top the toast and allow the juices of the tomato to soak into the bread.

385 calories

AVOCADO, FETA & MINT MASH

You may have been told that avocados are a no-no – nonsense, they're fantastic for you, taste like lovely green butter and fill you up for the day. Make a mash from ½ an avocado, a few cubes of feta and some freshly chopped mint, and spread liberally on your toast, cackling at your fanciness as you do.

427 calories

CHEESE & EGG

Rather than toasting your bread first, take each slice and, using your fists, gently make a well in the middle, then crack an egg into the well and sprinkle whatever cheese you like over the top (about 20g/¾ oz per slice). Pop under the grill until the cheese is browned and the yolk is still wobbly. Decorate with a few liberal drops of hot chilli sauce.

395 calories

PEANUT BUTTER & CARAMELIZED BANANA

Slice your banana and pop the slices into a non-stick pan – you're just browning them off a little – then pop them on top of peanut butter on toast. **Don't** use smooth peanut butter – not for any health reason, rather that it's simply disgusting.

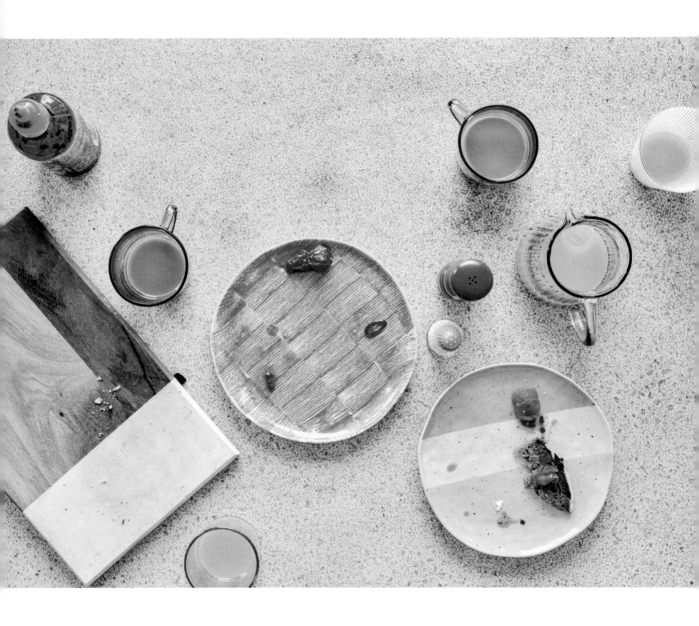

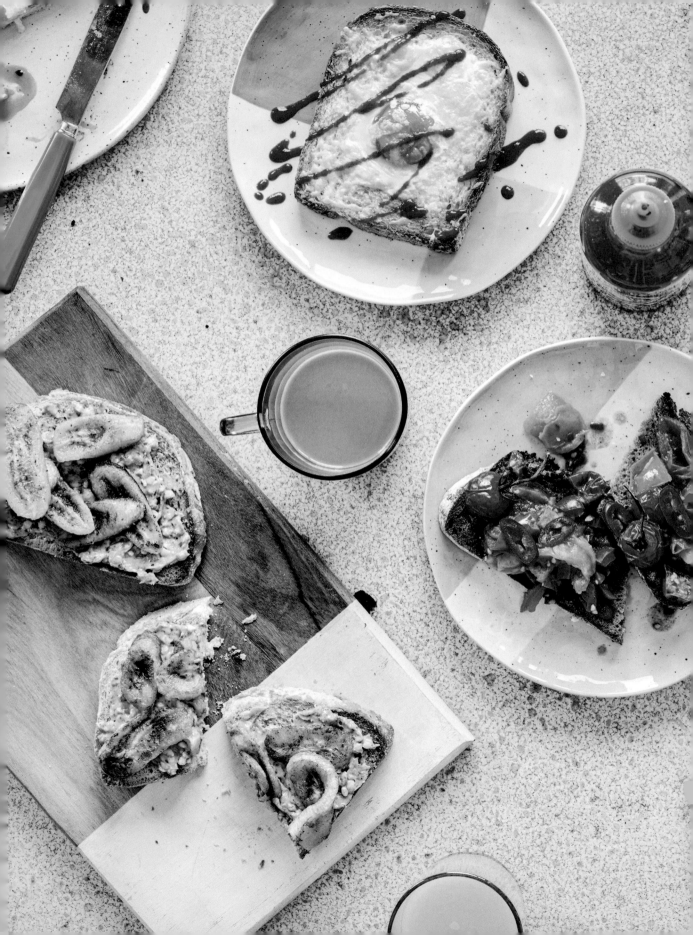

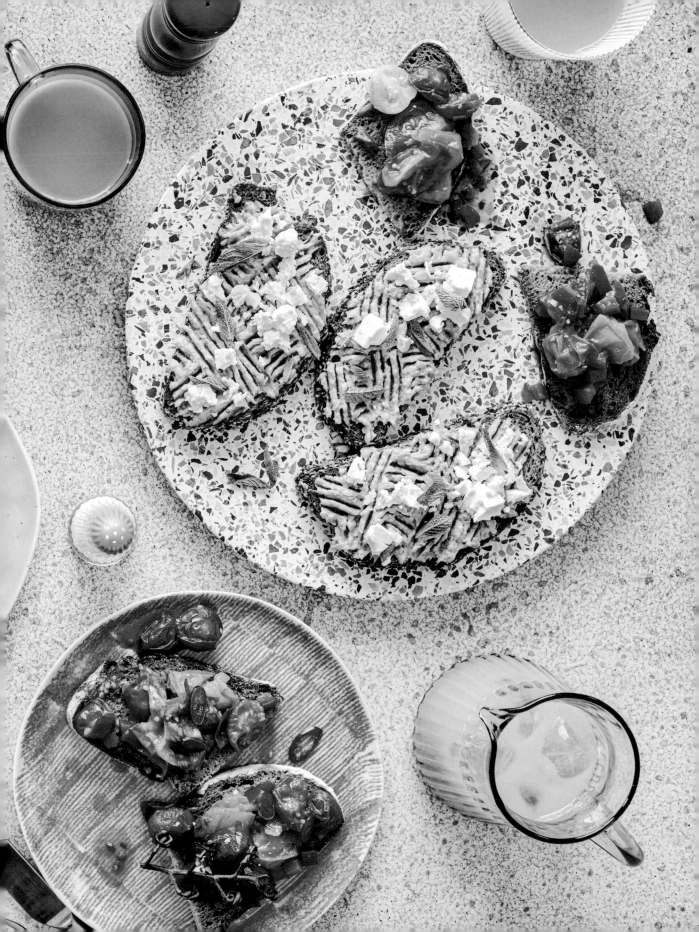

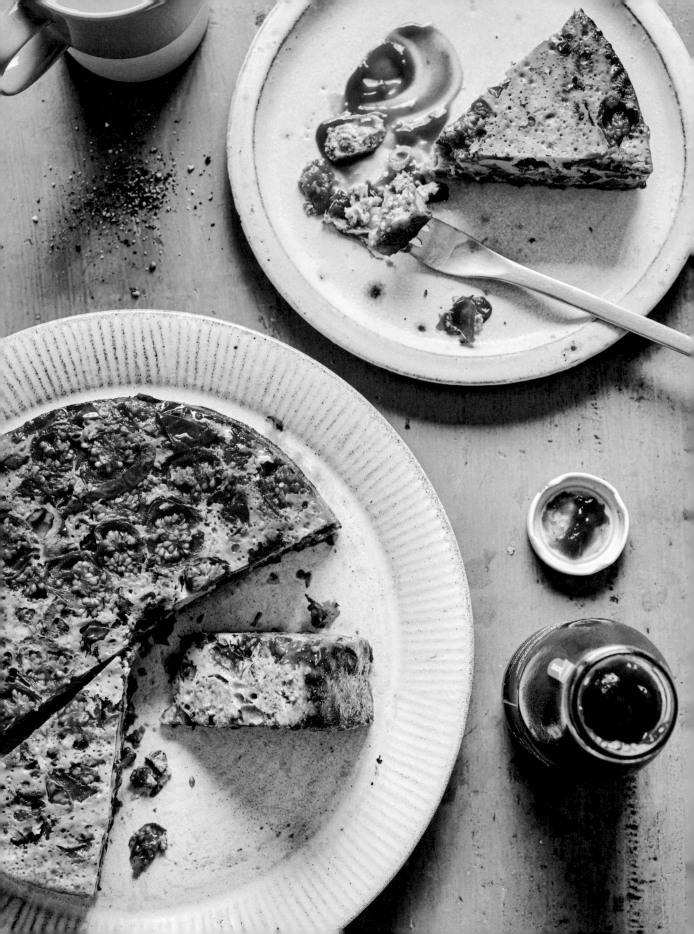

● ● ● ○ ● ●

FULL ENGLISH BREAKFAST QUICHE

Serves 4
498 calories

A reassuring wedge of quiche is a perfect start to the morning, and this wobbly beast is stuffed full of all the best bits of a full English breakfast. Topping it with slowly roasted chilli tomatoes may seem extravagant (and you'll note that we offer a quicker solution in the notes), but it will wake you up quicker than eight gallons of coffee ever will. As with all our recipes, feel free to add or subtract ingredients as you wish, though you'll struggle if you take out the eggs. Top tip: get yourself a 23cm (9 inch) deep-dish silicone cake tin for this. You can use your own dish if you have one, but getting the quiche out at the end will be an absolute doddle with silicone.

400g (14oz) cherry tomatoes
a pinch of chilli flakes
4 good-quality sausages, split open and the sausagemeat made into little tiny meatballs
110g (4oz) bacon lardons (or chop your own bacon if you're watching the fat content)
4 thick spring onions, sliced
200g (7oz/3 cups) button mushrooms, finely sliced
8 large eggs
50ml (2fl oz/¼ cup) milk
80g (3oz/¾ cup) grated mature Cheddar, grated
a pinch of sea salt and black pepper

Preheat your oven to 180°C fan/400°F/gas mark 6.

Slice your tomatoes in half, sprinkle with a pinch of chilli and sea salt, then spread them on a tray and pop them into the oven for 20 minutes, being careful not to let them char.

While the tomatoes are roasting, put the sausages, bacon, spring onions and mushrooms into a hot frying pan and cook until browned, making sure the water from the mushrooms has boiled away.

Take your tomatoes out of the oven when they've softened and mash them in a bowl.

Crack the eggs into a large bowl, add the milk, and whisk together with a good pinch of salt and pepper. Add the sausages, bacon, onions, mushrooms and cheese.

Spray the insides of your baking tin (see page 20) with low-fat cooking spray. Gently spoon the mashed tomatoes into the bottom of the tin and spread them around so you have a thin layer.

Carefully pour the quiche mix over the top – the gentler you are, the neater the results. No need to add cheese on the top of the quiche – you're going to flip this, so the 'top' of the quiche you can see at the moment will be the bottom.

Cover loosely with tin foil and bake for about 30 minutes, then remove the foil and bake for another 10 minutes, or until the eggs have set.

To serve, allow to cool, then it's time to be brave: place a plate on top of the dish, your hand underneath, and flip it – the quiche will drop out on to the plate and look at you, you've created a masterpiece!

Notes from Paul
- *Save time on the tomato front by simply reducing a tin of chopped tomatoes with some chilli and salt in a pan.*
- *Quiche is the best way to use up leftover allsorts from the fridge – don't be frightened to experiment.*

MEGA-EGGYBREAD CLUB SANDWICH STACKS

Serves 1
477 calories

2 slices of bread
1 tablespoon Dijon mustard
as much wafer-thin ham as you
    think you can get away with
    without an intervention
    (or about 35g/1oz)
same as above, but with wafer-
    thin chicken
1 large ripe tomato, sliced
slices of smoked cheese
2 eggs
salt and freshly ground black
    pepper

This is one of those recipes that lends itself to customization – add different meats, more cheese, peppers, more tomatoes, different mustards.

The key to this breakfast is making it the night before and wrapping it tight so everything sticks together – it'll make it so much easier when it comes to frying it towards the end. This makes enough for one sandwich, but as ever, scale up to satisfy your belly or dining partners.

We sometimes like to cut a large French stick in half lengthwise, pack in the fillings and wrap tightly as one long baguette – then, in the morning, we carefully cut slices and fry them as below.

Make up your sandwich – mustard on the bread, then layer the ham, chicken, sliced tomato and cheese as many times over as you want – we've managed 8 layers before now.

Wrap the sandwich as tightly as possible in clingfilm and pop it into the fridge – you want everything pressed together.

In the morning, take your sandwich out of the fridge. Beat the eggs with a pinch of salt and pepper and get your best frying pan out. Spray the pan with oil and set it over a medium heat.

Dip your sandwich into the egg mix, making sure it's coated and has soaked up as much as it can, then fry it. The ideal sandwich is one that is crispy on the outside and warm and gooey in the middle.

Serve with a side salad if you're still hungry, but I mean, come on …

Note from Paul
Add chilli flakes if you're one of those people who don't enjoy a meal without your lips burning.

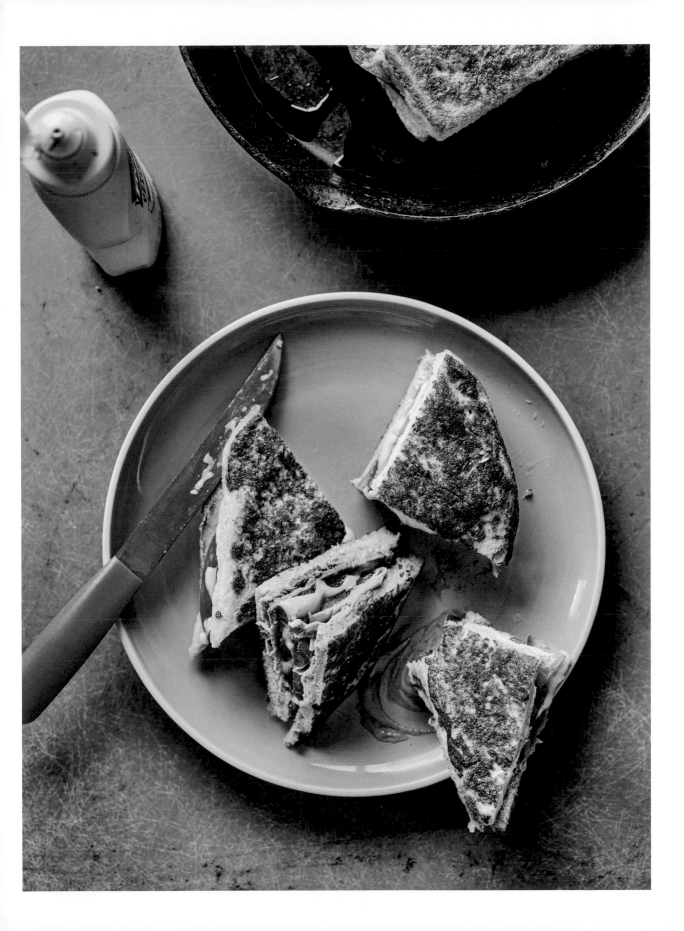

FIVE BASIC WAYS WITH AN EGG

Serves 1

191 calories for 2 eggs

239 calories
without any fillings

One thing we've noticed with slimming breakfasts is how many of them use eggs. If you're not a fan, then you're up the creek, and we apologise for your loss. You can do all manner of exciting things with eggs but sometimes the simplest things are the best, so here are the five basics.

We're lucky here at Chubby Towers – whenever we visit my parents, we leave laden with enough eggs to keep us going for forty years. My mum has taken to keeping chickens in her allotments and not a visit goes by without a twenty-minute update on how her hens are laying, what food she has been feeding them and what names she has decided to give them. It's all so breathtakingly exhilarating that we're thinking about putting her in a home early to celebrate.

Not everyone is blessed enough to have parents with such a fervent ovoid obsession, and if that's the case with you, just a couple of simple pleas. Get the best eggs you can afford – free-range at a minimum, stolen from the side of the road at best. Don't keep your eggs in the fridge (especially when making boiled eggs) – get yourself a fashionable metal cock to keep them in. It's what we use. Yep: cock.

HOW TO BOIL AN EGG

This might seem simple, but how many of us have boiled an egg, prepared our soldiers and then been met with abject disappointment at an egg you could use as a cricket ball – honestly, it keeps me awake at night.

Get your water boiling in a small pan and gently lower your eggs in with a spoon, as gently as you can, so they don't bounce off each other and crack. We go for 6 minutes for a dippy egg and 9 minutes for a hard-boiled egg.

As soon as you take the egg out of the boiling water, pop them into cold water to stop them cooking!

YOUR BASIC OMELETTE

Whisk 2 eggs together in a jug. Spray a good non-stick frying pan with a few spritzes of oil and heat to a medium heat.

Once the pan is warm, slowly tip in the egg mixture and gently tilt the pan to make sure the bottom is covered.

You'll know it's time to fold when the omelette can slide around on its own and the edges are cooked. Add your fillings to one half of the omelette, then fold the other half over using a fish-slice, or, if you're like me, your asbestos fingers.

Cook for another 2 minutes or so, especially if you have cheese in there so it goes gooey.

Note from Paul
Before you tip the egg mixture in, fry some very thinly sliced onions and then pour the egg over the top – omelette with fried onions baked right in!

PERFECT (CHEATING) POACHED EGGS

149 calories for 2 eggs

We can't poach an egg the traditional way to save our lives – we managed it once and then never again, like finding a four-leaf clover or monogamy.

So, we cheat: get a small bowl, fill it with cold water and crack the egg into it. Microwave for around 45 seconds. Take the egg out with a slotted spoon.

Now this does have the rather unfortunate side-effect of giving you an egg like a McDonalds 'egg', but just own your slattery and make a joke about it.

SCRAMBLED EGGS

294 calories

Whisk together 2 eggs with a splash of milk and a pinch of salt.

Pour the mixture into a frying pan and add a drop or 2 of oil.

Two choices here: either keep whisking as it sets, to get fluffy eggs, or let it cook a bit and dice towards the end for more 'ribbony' eggs.

Don't cook it until it's completely set – it'll keep cooking long after you remove it from the heat, so factor that in unless you want eggs with the texture of a seat cushion.

We add a load of chives and cheese to our scrambled eggs because, frankly, such a simple thing can never go unadorned in our lives.

BAKED EGGS

258 calories

Nice and simple this one – you just need a tiny ovenproof dish. Those ramekins from fancy desserts work well.

Layer the bottom of the ramekin with whatever you fancy – chopped ham, tomatoes, mushrooms, passata, beans – then crack 2 eggs on top.

Bake in the oven at around 180°C fan/400°F/gas mark 6, until the egg has set firm.

LOCO MOCO

Serves 4
494 calories

Bit of a tenuous one, this – for our honeymoon so many moons ago, we stayed at Disney's Polynesian Resort. It was fantastic, even if I did make a faux pas with £1 sun cream from a budget shop which turned me blue. Nothing says 'take me to bed and make me an honest woman' like looking like an oxygen-deprived Smurf. Nevertheless, we ate like kings, and one of our fondest memories from the Polynesian was a breakfast called loco moco, which, put simply, is beef on rice topped with an egg. The idea of having mince and rice for breakfast might seem peculiar but this is actually quite a light dish so don't be afraid. Having said that, it works just as well as an evening meal. See the notes if you need to speed this up!

200g (7oz/1 cup) white rice
300g (10½oz) lean beef mince
     (keeping the fat content down
     if you're slimming)
4 large eggs
instant gravy – and don't be
     stingy here, get the good stuff!
3 red and green chillies, finely
     diced, for the top
a good pinch of salt and freshly
     ground black pepper

Give your rice a good rinse under cold water and then get it boiling until it's cooked through – we follow the '1 rice, 2 water' rule – if you're using a cup of rice, use 2 cups of water, but always keep an eye on it.

Meanwhile, get your mince and take all your frustration out on it, kneading and squeezing it and then forming it into 4 equal-sized burgers – make sure to season each side liberally with salt and pepper.

Fry the burgers in a good non-stick pan with a few sprays of olive oil until cooked through, then pop to one side, keeping the pan hot.

Crack the eggs into the pan and cook them however you like your eggs in the morning – we like ours with a kiss (and the yolks runny enough to dip in).

Once the rice is cooked and drained, the eggs perfect and the burgers seared, get assembling – rice, burger, egg – then slather lovingly with the gravy and top with the diced chillies.

Notes from Paul
- *You can make this into a super quick breakfast by using a pouch of microwave rice (and if you do, we recommend a coconut-flavoured edition) and a decent pre-shaped burger.*
- *If you're not a fan of sweating profusely on the morning commute, maybe leave the chillies off.*

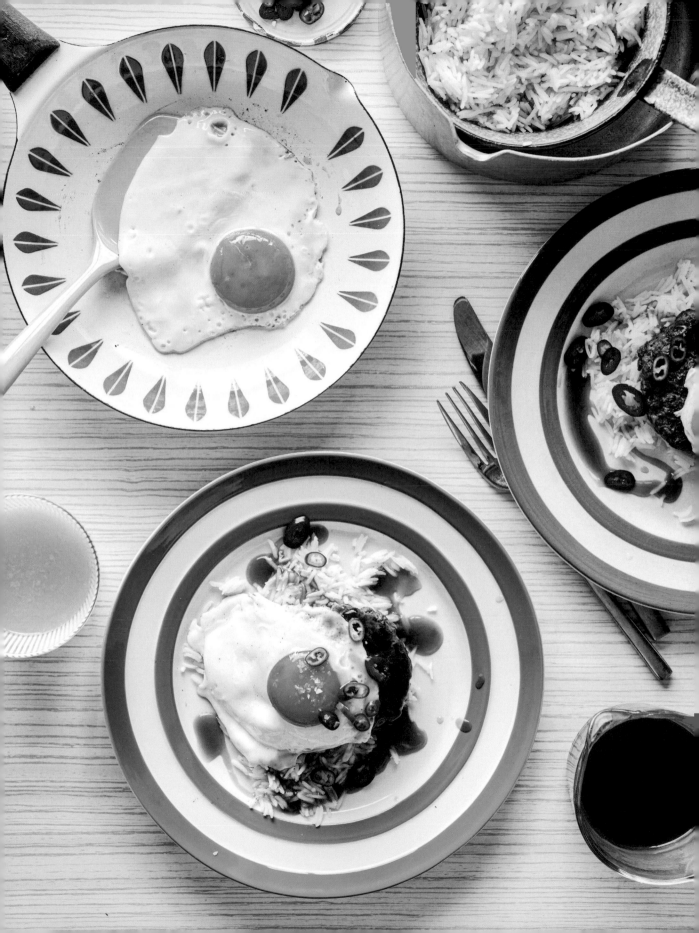

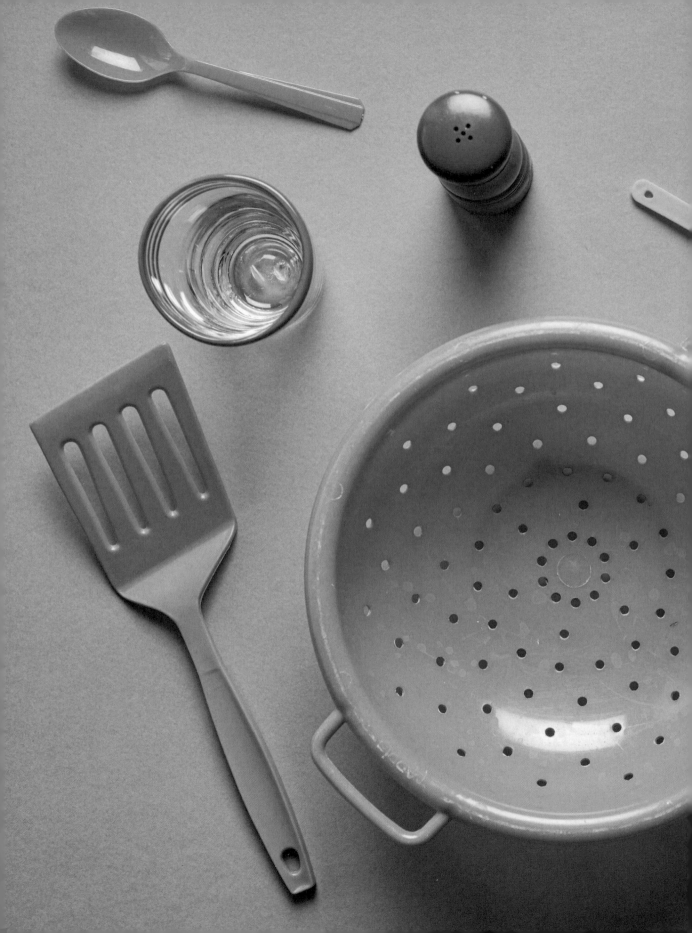

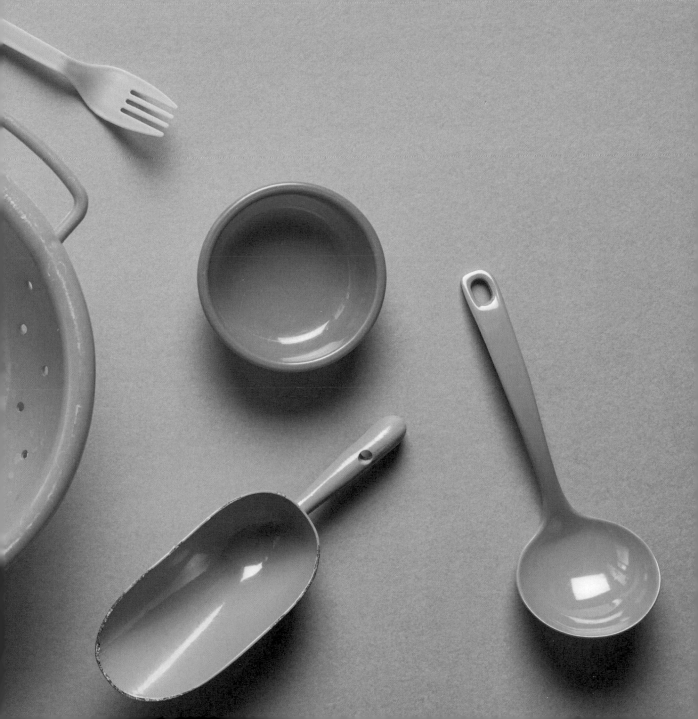

LUNCH & LIGHT BITES

GRANNY'S GARDEN FRITTATA

Serves 4
116 calories

We're calling this Granny's garden frittata simply because my nana, to whom the book is dedicated, spent her days pottering around in her garden. She was always especially proud of the vegetables that she managed to cultivate, even if she did then cook them in so much salt that you would be forgiven for thinking she had dredged them out of the sea.

Now, listen – you know we encourage mixing things up with our recipes, and really, there couldn't be a better recipe than this to try that out on. We went with whatever we could find in our freezer that wasn't vodka, and it worked a treat, but recipes like this can carry anything.

This is a great vegetarian recipe – the inclusion of goat's cheese may give you a moment of pause but it really mustn't – we have been reassured that you can get vegetarian goat's cheese. What a time to be alive. If you're not a fan of cheese that smells like a decomposed foot, simply swap it for Edam or Gouda.

75g (2¾oz) courgettes, sliced
90g (3¼oz) trimmed asparagus, cut into 1cm (½ inch) chunks
70g (2½oz/1 cup) mushrooms, sliced
1 clove of garlic, crushed
50g (1¾oz) spinach
3 eggs
50ml (2 fl oz/¼ cup) milk
50g (1¾/¼ cup) goat's cheese
freshly ground black pepper

You'll need a frying pan that can withstand going under the grill. Spray the pan with a little oil, add the sliced courgette and the asparagus chunks, and cook over a medium heat until they soften.

Add the mushrooms, garlic and spinach, give it all a stir, and cover the pan with a lid until the spinach has wilted.

Beat the eggs and milk in a jug until frothy, adding black pepper as you go, then pour over the veg. Crumble the goat's cheese on top and cook for a few minutes, until the frittata is almost set with just a wee wobble in the middle.

Finish it off under the grill for a couple of minutes until everything is set and toasty.

Notes from Paul
- Sliced yellow peppers work well here, as do thinly sliced potatoes, if you would like to make this into more of a Spanish omelette (you fancy soul).
- Be careful about adding tomatoes – they're delicious, but the added liquid might make your frittata moist, and goodness knows we don't want that.
- This keeps superbly well in the fridge, so keep a slice for a next-day lunch.

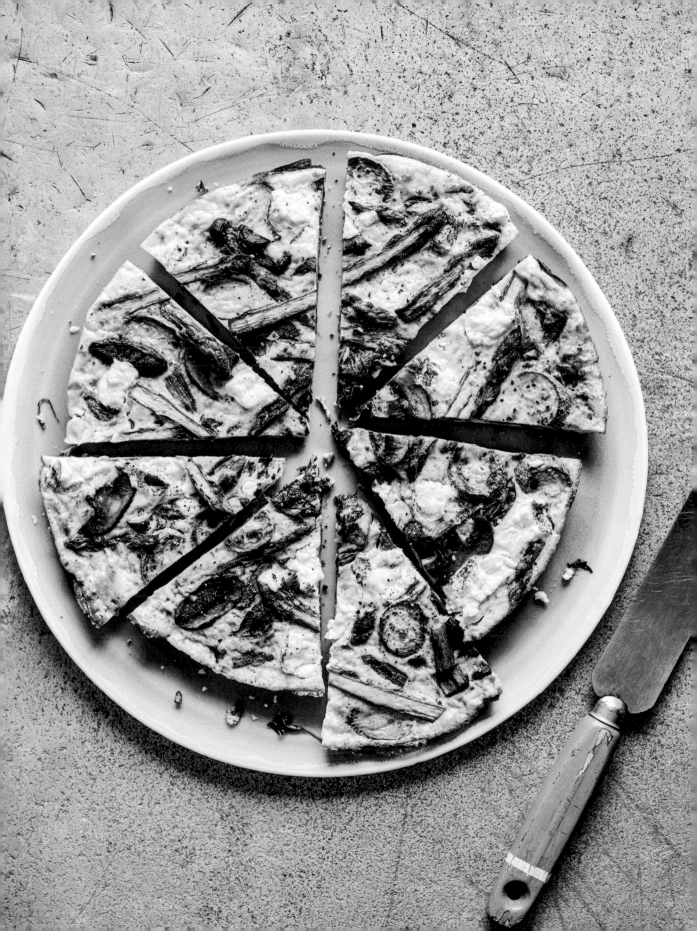

A RIGHT NICE MINESTRONE SOUP

Serves 4
498 calories

When you're poorly sick and feeling sorry for yourself, a proper bowl of good soup is exactly what you need. This soup is exactly that – not fancy, not exciting, just good old-fashioned medicine in a bowl.

I don't cope well with being unwell. In fact, I was going to launch into a couple of tales of nonsense about being a terrible patient to Paul's Florence Nightingale routine (he needs a bloody big girdle to get into that nurse's outfit) but instead, I'm popping my serious hat on.

I've talked on the blog about my battles with anxiety and how I spent years of my life convinced I was about to die. I always try to tell people that it can get better, though I never believed it when people said it to me (even my own doctor), but hey, it might just hit home for one of you. Do take a look at my stories online to see the progression of my illness and how I overcame it – it'll keep you chipper.

And you really, really ought to try this soup. If anything, cutting up the vegetables will keep your mind occupied and, as a very wise man once said to me, busy hands stop a busy mind. Tis true, that.

160g (5¾oz) bacon, finely diced
4 cloves of garlic, finely chopped
1 large onion, finely diced
200g (7oz/1½ cups) fennel, finely diced
1 red chilli, finely sliced
a handful of fresh basil leaves
1 large carrot, finely diced
250g (9oz/2 cups) celery stalks, finely diced
1 × 400g (14oz) tin of chopped tomatoes
1 large potato, peeled and diced into small cubes
1 × 400g (14oz) tin of butter beans, drained
2 vegetable stock cubes
150g (5½oz/1 cup) fresh or frozen peas
1 large courgette, finely diced
1 red pepper, finely diced
200g (7oz/2 cups) wholemeal soup pasta

Heat a large saucepan over a medium-high heat and spray with some oil. Add the bacon and fry for 2–3 minutes.

Add the garlic, onion and fennel and cook for another 2 minutes, then add the chilli, basil, carrot and celery. Give it a good stir, then reduce the heat a little and leave to cook for another 5 minutes.

Add the chopped tomatoes and the potato, stir, and cook for another 10 minutes. Give another stir and simmer for 5 more minutes.

Add the butter beans and a litre (1¾ pints/ 4cups of boiling water, and crumble in the stock cubes. Add the peas, courgettes and peppers. Give it a stir, then cover with a lid and leave to simmer for 10–15 minutes. Remove from the heat and allow to rest for 15 minutes or so.

Cook the pasta according to the packet instructions. Add the drained pasta to the soup and serve.

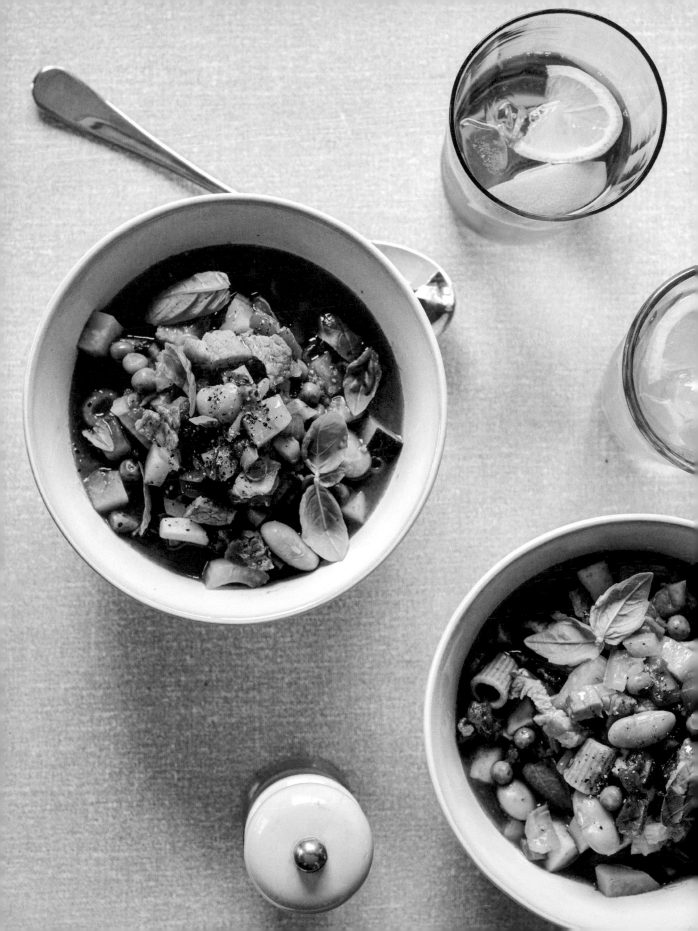

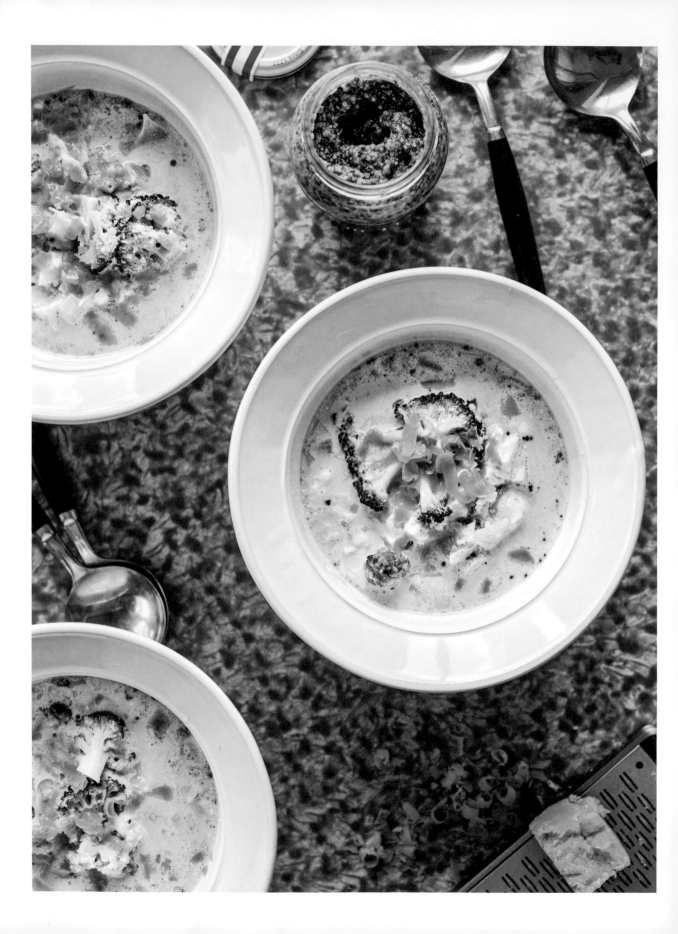

● ● ● ● ● ●

SLOW-COOKED CHEESY BROCCOLI SOUP

Serves 4
170 calories

200g (7oz) cauliflower florets
280g (10oz) broccoli florets, chopped
750ml (1 ¼ pints/3 cups) chicken stock
3 cloves of garlic
1 onion, diced
1 teaspoon wholegrain mustard
1 teaspoon salt
¼ teaspoon freshly ground black pepper
100g (3½oz/½ cup) extra-light soft cheese
60g (2oz/½ cup) reduced-fat Red Leicester cheese, grated, to serve

I have my mother to thank for a lot of things: my liberal use of profanity, my messed-up nose (I went arse-over-teakettle on a bike ride once, landed on my nose, was treated with a tea-towel and lots of tutting) and my ability to shave – I always wanted a 'tache like hers, growing up. However, we ought to give credit where it's due and show our appreciation for this soup: it's one of her recipes, though I've tinkered with it just enough to remove the cigarette ash.

I tease my mother an awful lot on the blog and I daresay regular readers have this image of her as some workhouse scrubber with a filthy mouth and a cruel, malevolent streak. That's incredibly unfair: she's actually been the perfect mother to me, and lord knows I put her through a lot.

The original recipe has been changed somewhat: Mother liked to use blue cheese and cream rather than soft cheese and Red Leicester, for example. But see, blue cheese is altogether too divisive in Chubby Towers: I can't get enough of it, but Paul thinks it looks and smells like a sweaty bum. However, if you're feeling especially decadent – and mind, when aren't you? – go right ahead and change it up. Paul suggests that this can be done in a slow cooker and perhaps it could, but honestly, a pan will do just fine and means you're not coming back to a house that smells entirely of farts.

Blitz the cauliflower florets in a food processor or grate with a cheese grater until they resemble rice.

Place all the ingredients except for the cheese in a large pan and gently simmer for 1 hour.

Add the soft cheese and stir well.

Serve the soup in bowls, sprinkled with the grated cheese.

Note from Paul
This will work well in the slow cooker! Follow the same instructions as above, but cook on low for 8 hours.

FIVE SANDWICH FILLINGS

Each filling makes 1 sandwich (serves 1)

I don't know about you, but sandwiches for me are a real treat and proper comfort food. When I was a kid my dad once took me to Wicksteed Park and packed up some lovely egg and salad cream sandwiches, my favourite. He even used proper butter! Of course, being a fatty, on the way home I spotted an errant sandwich that had fallen down the back, still wrapped up, so I thought, why the hell not? I unwrapped it and the unholiest stench came out. Not to be beaten, I ate the whole thing and I reckon it probably sat in my gut for no more than eight minutes before I was begging my dad to pull over on the side of the A605 so I could lose all dignity. Needless to say it hasn't put me off. Sandwiches are still my fave, even those that have sat on the back seat of a hot Renault 19 for five hours …

366 calories

CORONATION CHICKEN (see page 60)

Mix together about 70g (2½oz) diced, cooked, skinless chicken breast with a few teaspoons of reduced-fat mayonnaise. Add a teaspoon of mango chutney and a pinch of curry powder for flavouring, and sprinkle in a few sultanas.

369 calories

CHEESE SAVOURY (opposite)

Chop up some onions and peppers, and grate a little bit of carrot. Sprinkle in 40g (1½oz/¼ cup) grated cheese, mixed with a bit of reduced-fat mayo.

322 calories

TUNA CRUNCH (see page 59)

Get together some of your best chopped salad ingredients – peppers, onions, cucumbers all go well in this. Mix with a drained tin of tuna, and drizzle in a little balsamic vinegar for some sass.

389 calories

EGG SALAD (see page 58)

A classic, but a goodie! Boil a couple of eggs for 10 minutes, rinse under cold water and peel. Mash with a fork (no need to be dainty), and chuck in either a little bit of reduced-fat mayonnaise or, my favourite, salad cream. Add some cress and sliced spring onions.

365 calories

CHINESE CHICKEN (see page 61)

Cook some chicken in a slow cooker or pressure cooker and shred. Once cooled, mix with a little hoisin sauce and natural yoghurt, and sprinkle in a little five-spice along with some chunks of cucumber and spring onion.

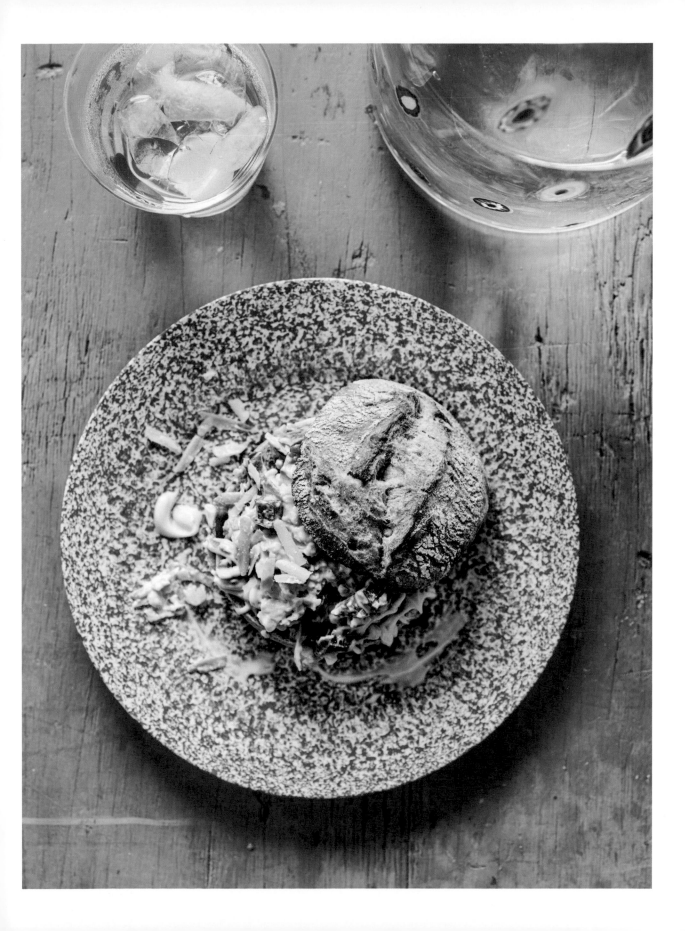

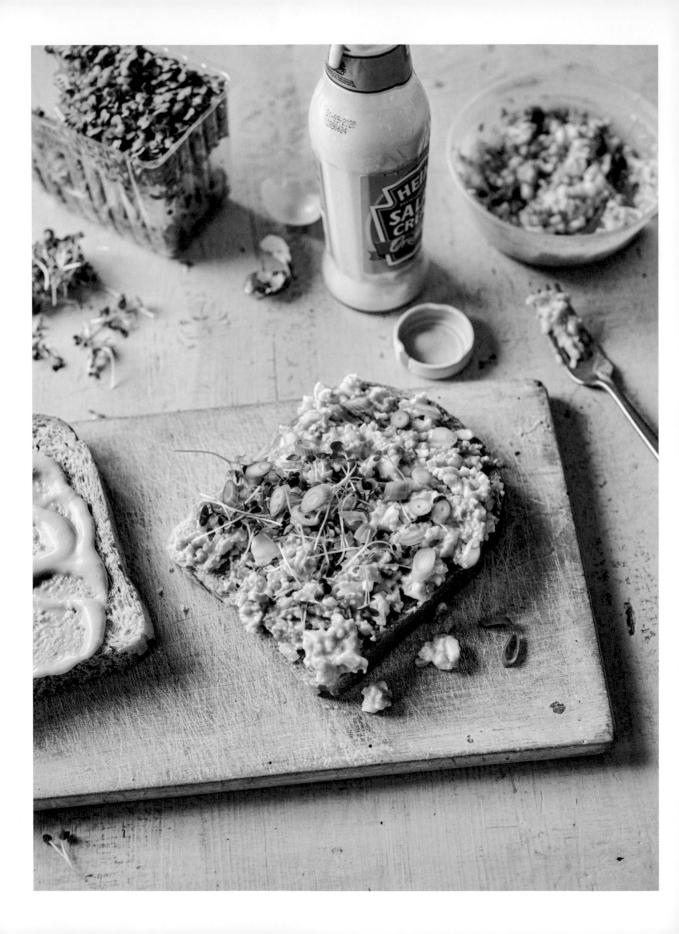

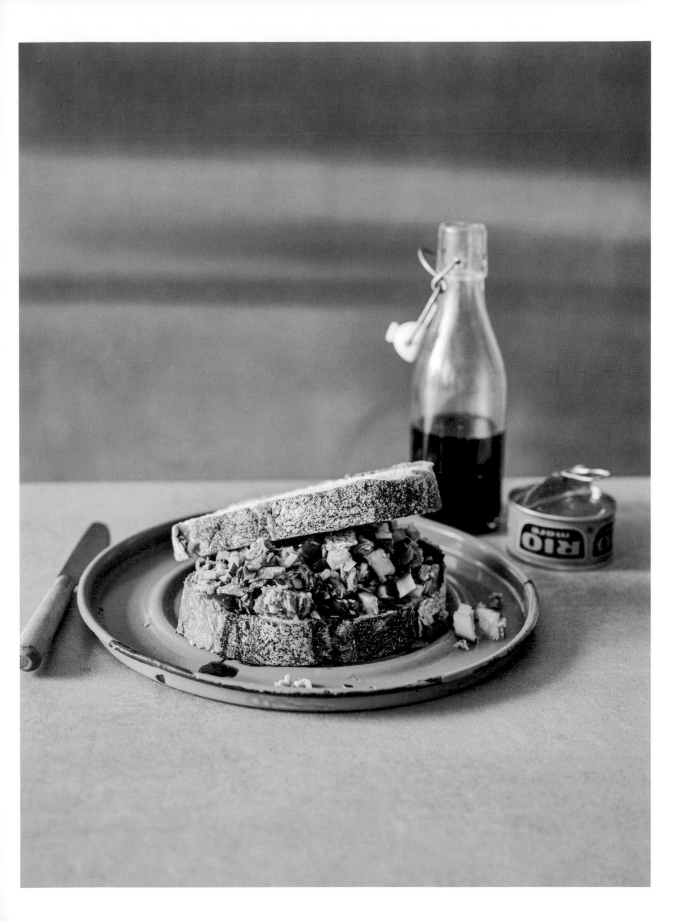

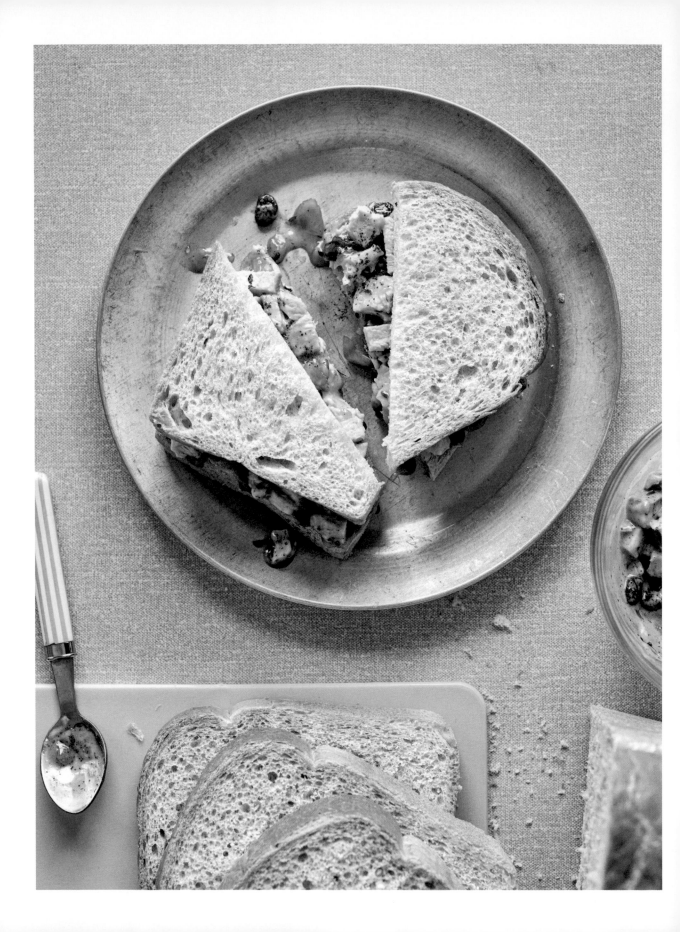

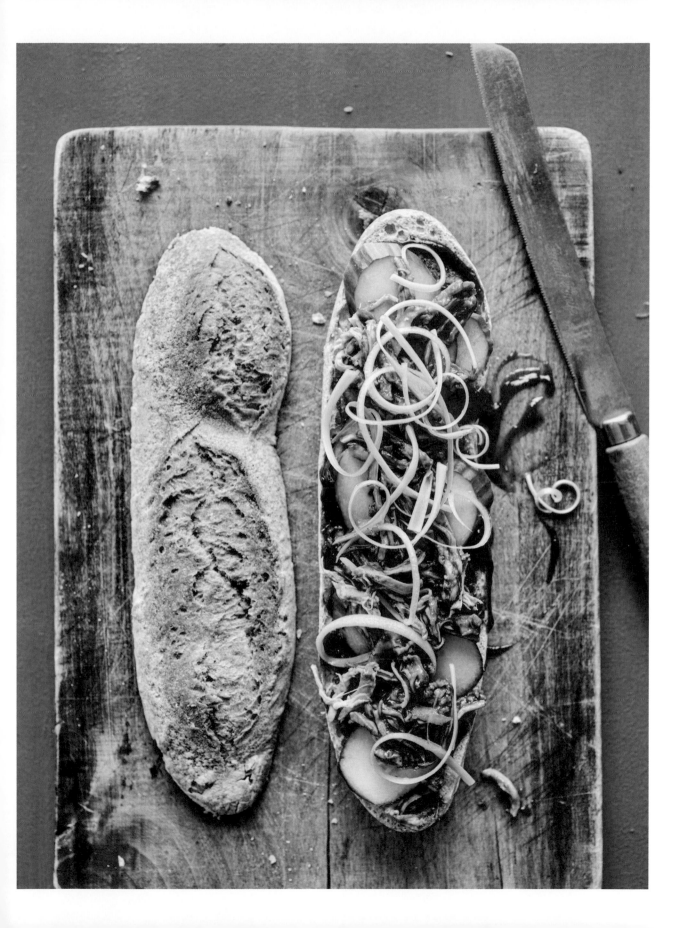

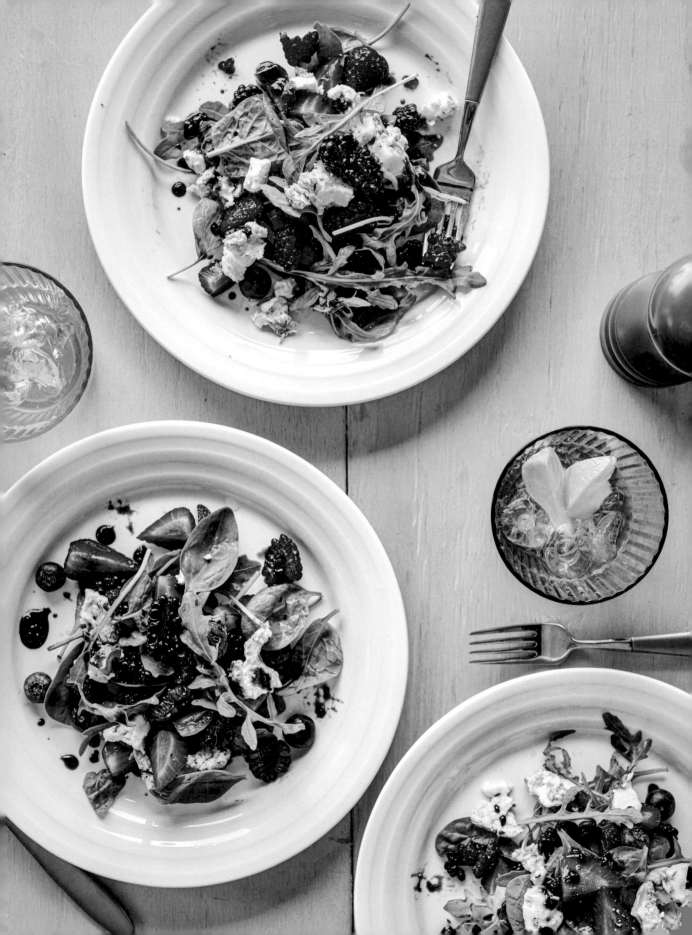

BERRY BERRY SALAD

Serves 4
132 calories

We previously lived in the centre of Newcastle in a fancy, definitely-not-sticking-the-rent-on-a-credit-card apartment. It was terribly exciting and a great place to live as two young men exploring our bodies and finding our way in the world. However, Paul, with his subscription to Subterranean Exploration monthly (neither a joke nor a euphemism, sadly) and books on concrete, decided that we needed to move somewhere a little more sedate. So we did, into the land that time forgot. We now have a charming bungalow that previously belonged to one careful old lady owner (who promptly died on the toilet, so we also have a haunted bathroom) and it's ideal (though I did have to fight Paul to get the commode taken out).

One advantage of Chubby Towers is that it comes with altogether more garden than we know what to do with. When we moved in I had grand plans of turning the back into a proper produce garden, keeping the blog going with whimsical posts about what vegetables were in season. Like Penelope Keith in The Good Life, only dressed in slacks from George at ASDA. This grand plan started well – I cleared the soil, had some planters built from railway sleepers, bought a pipe to smoke luxuriously while I tilled the earth. Then I realized that gardening involves bending over and working up a sweat, and frankly that's not for me. So I chucked a few bee bombs at the soil and now we have wildflowers growing everywhere. It's marvellous, actually (and we must save the bees!) and I heartily recommend everyone does the same.

However, the one thing I have managed to keep alive is a charming little blackberry bush hidden round the back of my greenhouse. I can only assume it's so I can dash through the barbed branches and feel alive. A steamy summer a couple of years ago produced an overabundance of berries and so they made it into this salad. Not a fan of a particular berry? That's fine: swap them out for whatever you like. Any leftover fruit can be honeyed and used to top some toast – see our recipe on page 36.

125ml (4fl oz/½ cup) balsamic vinegar
100g (3½oz/1 cup) raspberries
140g (5oz) rocket
140g (5oz) baby leaf spinach
200g (7oz/2 cups) strawberries, quartered
100g (3½oz/1 cup) blackberries
50g (1¾oz/½ cup) blueberries
90g (3¼oz/¾ cup) goat's cheese, crumbled

Put the balsamic vinegar into a small saucepan together with 40g (1½oz/⅓ cup) of raspberries and bring to the boil, mashing the raspberries a little to break them down.

Reduce the heat and simmer for 10 minutes, stirring occasionally, then remove from the heat and allow to cool.

Gently toss together the rocket, spinach, the remaining raspberries and other berries, and serve on 4 plates.

Top with the crumbled goat's cheese, and drizzle with the raspberry vinegar.

●●●●●●

CRUNCHY MUNCHY WALDORF SALAD

Serves 4
248 calories

150g (5½oz/1 cup) black grapes
50g (1½oz/¼ cup) walnuts
2 tablespoons reduced-fat
   mayonnaise
200g (7oz/1 cup) fat-free yoghurt
½ teaspoon mustard powder
juice of 1 lemon
1 romaine lettuce, roughly
   chopped
2 apples, sliced into matchsticks
2 celery stalks, cut into 1cm
   (½ inch) thick slices

We had our first Waldorf salad back in 2016, in some fabulously expensive hotel in New York. I had surprised Paul with a last-minute getaway – literally didn't tell him where we were going until we turned up at the airport and picked up our boarding passes.

I tend to pick the places we'll eat when away on holiday because I love nothing more than researching, poring over menus and then getting somewhere and deciding on something entirely different. As part of the 'surprise' holiday, I gave Paul carte blanche to choose our destinations.

He chose a TGI Fridays. On Times Square. Now, listen: there's nothing wrong with a TGI Fridays, absolutely not. But for context, we have two within a fifteen minute drive of our house. New York has over 25,000 restaurants, and Paul chose that. I believe we paid almost $115 for two Chef-Ding burgers, a couple of cocktails and a dessert so gloopy I'm still, even now, trying to brush it through my chest hair. The worst part? Because this was a surprise holiday and an act of love, I couldn't even express my frustration and instead had to sit with an obsequious rictus grin throughout. Not that I've held onto this, you understand …

This salad more than made up for that little disaster, however. If you're not a fan of the walnuts you could absolutely leave them out, but then you wouldn't have a Waldorf salad. You could leave out the lettuce and replace with chips if you prefer, but see, that's why we are where we are right now.

Preheat the oven to 180°C fan/400°F/gas mark 6.

Place the grapes on a baking tray and spray them with a little oil. Cook them in the oven for 10 minutes, then add the walnuts and cook for another 5 minutes. Remove them from the oven.

In a bowl mix together the mayonnaise, yoghurt and mustard powder and squeeze in the lemon juice.

Mix the lettuce, apple and celery in a large bowl, then gently mix in the grapes. Chop the walnuts roughly and add them to the bowl. Pour over the yoghurt mixture, stir gently and serve.

Notes from Paul

- We like romaine lettuce because it's got a bit of bite, but feel free to use whatever lettuce you like.
- Roasting the grapes and the walnuts adds to the flavour, but if you're stuck for time you can put them both in as they are.
- If you haven't got any mustard powder you can use 1 tablespoon of mustard instead – wholegrain is best.

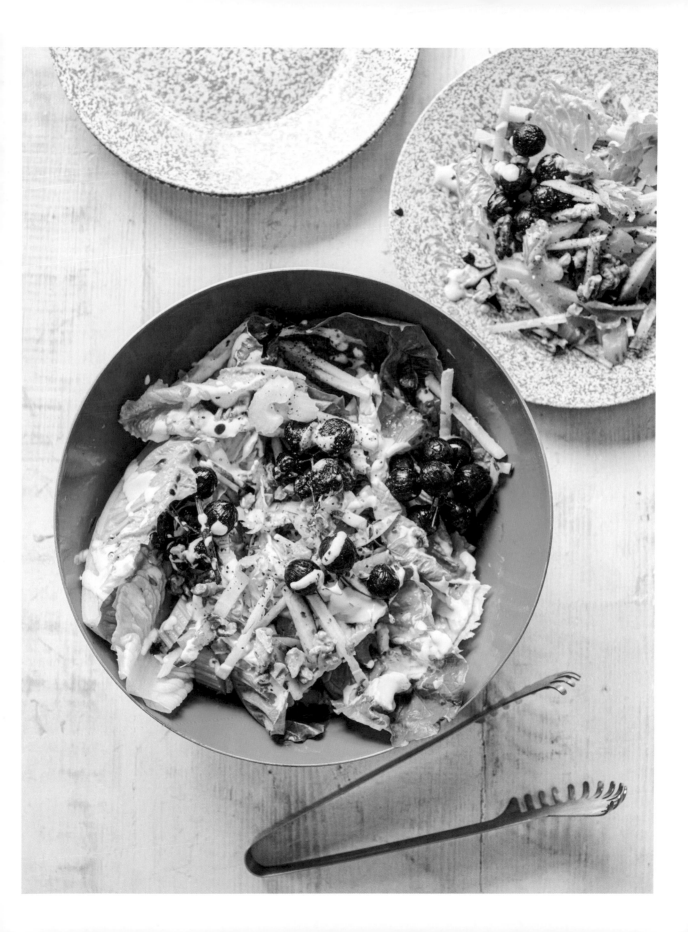

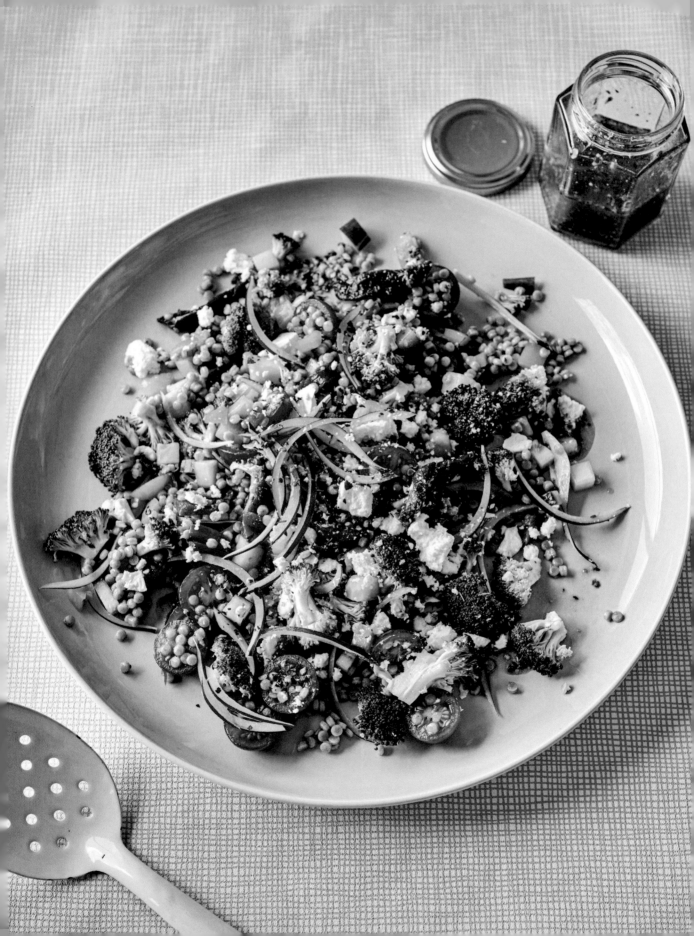

• • • • • •

CHOPPED COUSCOUS SALAD

Serves 4
301 calories

This is the perfect dish for a trip in the car, if you're one of those sensible folks who can have a picnic basket full of goodies in the back and have the restraint not to crack it open by time you've backed off the drive.

Car journeys in the Twochubbycubs world are always an especially fraught affair. It's a long running joke that if I'm driving then it'll take four times as long to get there because I like to stop at every single service station in case I miss something exciting. If Paul is driving, he still loses. See: I am an absolutely awful passenger. Every single journey results in the same arguments about his music (dreadful), driving ability (sub-par compared to mine) and awful car (who buys a car the size of a rollerskate?).

You know, the more I write this book, the more I realize what a bum's rush Paul gets from this marriage. QUICK: DISTRACTION – TO THE RECIPE BEFORE HE REALISES! SOMETHING ABOUT COUSCOUS, YES YES.

120g (4oz/1 cup) wholewheat giant couscous
300g (10½oz) cherry tomatoes, halved
6 sun-dried tomatoes, chopped
1 red onion, sliced
1 small head of broccoli, chopped into tiny florets
½ a cucumber, sliced
a couple of large roasted peppers (from a jar)
1 yellow pepper, chopped
160g (5¾oz/1 cup) reduced-fat feta cheese, crumbled

For the vinaigrette
60ml (2fl oz/¼ cup) red wine vinegar
1 tablespoon olive oil
2 teaspoons wholegrain mustard
1 tablespoon honey
1 tablespoon lemon juice
1 teaspoon dried mixed herbs
½ teaspoon salt
¼ teaspoon freshly ground black pepper
a pinch of crushed chilli flakes

Mix together the vinaigrette ingredients and set aside.

Bring a saucepan of water to the boil and add the couscous. Stir, cover with the lid, and simmer for 6–8 minutes, then drain and allow to cool.

Mix the couscous with the rest of the salad ingredients and serve, drizzled with the vinaigrette.

Notes from Paul
· If you can't find giant couscous, regular couscous will work just as well.
· For a healthier option, try to use dehydrated sun-dried tomatoes rather than the ones in oil – all they need is 10 minutes in hot water to plump up.
· Not a fan of crunchy broccoli? We understand – chuck the bigger florets in with the couscous when you cook it, to soften.

● ● ● ● ● ●

CHEESY CHUBBY FISHCAKES

Serves 4
358 calories

400g (14oz) cod or haddock
150ml (5fl oz/⅔ cup) milk
150ml (5fl oz/⅔ cup) water
400g (14oz) potatoes, peeled
2 eggs
a small bunch of fresh chives,
    chopped
100g (3½oz/1 cup) Gruyère, diced
80g (3oz/1 cup) panko
    breadcrumbs
salt

We absolutely adore these fishcakes, which is surprising as neither of us can bear fish as a rule. However, turns out if you add some crunchy breadcrumbs and more than a decent amount of cheese, it can be made quite palatable.

Inspiration for this recipe came from my sheer determination to make a fishcake that went far beyond the orange and grey pucks of 'fish' that we used to get served at school, and I rather think we've nailed it with these.

Place the fish in a frying pan and add the milk and water. Bring to the boil, then reduce the heat and simmer for 3–4 minutes.

Remove the pan from the heat, cover with a lid and leave to sit for 10 minutes. Lift the fish out of the pan and set aside.

Meanwhile, chop the potatoes into cubes a few centimetres (about an inch) across, and place in a large saucepan. Cover with water, add a pinch of salt, bring to the boil, then reduce the heat and simmer for 10 minutes, or until the potatoes are tender.

Drain the potatoes and tip them back into the pan. Break in 1 egg and mash the potatoes quickly.

Gently break the fish up into large chunks with a fork and drop it into the mash together with the chopped chives and the cheese. Gently mix with a spoon, being careful not to break the fish up too much.

Beat the remaining egg and pour it into a shallow dish, and put the panko into another shallow dish. Divide the mash mixture into 4 and squash each one into a burger shape. Gently dip each one into the egg mix and then into the panko, making sure to coat the entire fishcake.

Spray a large frying pan with a little oil and carefully fry the fishcakes for 4–5 minutes on each side, until golden.

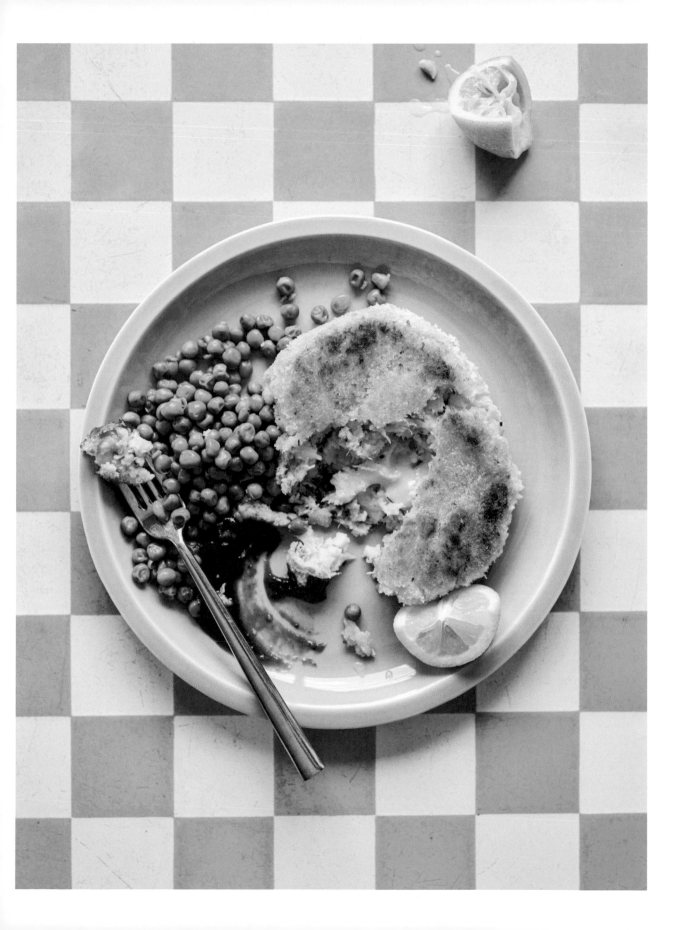

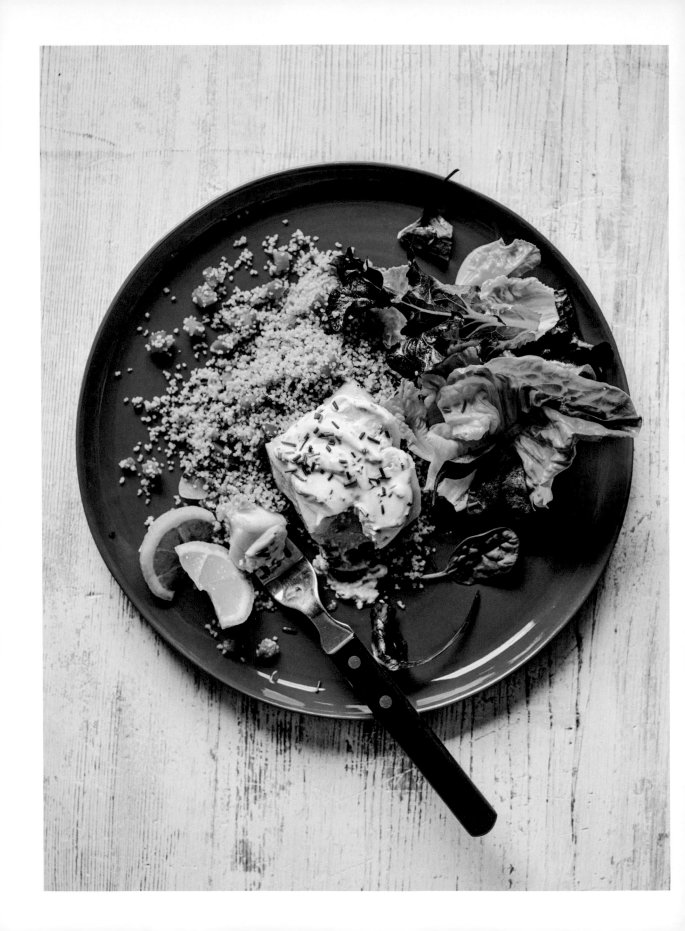

• • • • • •

LEMON COD
WITH COUSCOUS

Serves 4
472 calories

Of all the places in the world to source recipe inspiration, would you have ever thought the NHS – that wonderful bastion of all things excellent and wonderful – would be one of ours? But it is! I've only had cause to stay over in hospital twice in my life – one when I performed a partial circumcision on myself in my haste to pull my zip up and get back to the office buffet, the other when I was much smaller and had to get my tongue 'untied'. Even now I can see that my mother remains haunted by that decision, suffered as she has through the resulting years of me never shutting the hell up.

I was never served this lemon cod and couscous as a patient – no, I was served this dish as a visitor. See, when Paul and I first started getting serious, he used to work in our local hospital as a records clerk. Given he was only a fifteen minute bus-ride away, I used to diligently get the bus over on a lunch time and 'see my man'. You might think that I was being romantic but, in fact, I just wanted to use his staff discount in the cafeteria – this being one the dishes that (despite my dislike of anything that swims) was worth enduring his fascinating administrative chat for.

Do try this recipe, it's a genuine delight. If you want to recreate the James and Paul story, liberally sprinkle your tablecloth with TCP and have a loved one sit opposite you talking about bladder surgery. It really lifts the dish!

420ml (15fl oz/1¾ cups) chicken stock
300g (10½oz/2 cups) couscous
100g (3½oz/¾ cup) carrots, finely diced
1 small onion, finely diced
2 cloves of garlic, crushed
½ teaspoon salt
½ teaspoon freshly ground black pepper
75ml (2½fl oz/⅓ cup) dry white wine
2 tablespoons reduced-fat Greek-style yoghurt
1 tablespoon lemon juice
2 tablespoons chopped fresh chives
4 cod fillets

Preheat the oven to 200°C fan/425°F/gas mark 7.

Pour the chicken stock into a saucepan and bring to the boil. Stir in the couscous, then cover with a lid and remove from the heat. Leave the couscous for 5–10 minutes, until all the liquid has been absorbed, then fluff with a fork.

Meanwhile, heat a large frying pan over a medium-high heat and spray with a little oil. Add the carrots, onion and garlic and cook for 5–6 minutes, stirring occasionally. Add the salt, pepper and wine and cook for another minute.

Add the cooked couscous and stir well, then cover with a lid and set aside.

Mix together the yoghurt, lemon juice and chives and spread over the top of the cod fillets.

Heat a large ovenproof frying pan over a high heat and spray with a little oil. Add the cod to the pan, yoghurt-side up, and cook for 2–3 minutes. Transfer the pan to the oven and bake for 5–7 minutes, until cooked.

Serve the couscous on plates and top each one with a cod fillet.

PROPER HAM & EGG QUICHE

Serves 4
310 calories

On a diet, there's absolutely no way of having a quiche with thick buttery pastry. Well, no, there is – a little of everything in moderation, after all. But none of us got to the point where we struggle to see our feet by eating in moderation. We've seen many fads come and go – bread wraps, cottage cheese and pease pudding, to name three – but they never quite hit the spot.

So, not going to fib here, we usually use pastry, and then feel bad about ourselves afterwards. Until we have more. But this take on a ham and egg quiche proved wildly popular despite the lack of pastry, and the sweet potato creates a base to hold everything in place. It's not going to leave you with pastry crumbs all down your front, no, but it'll sure fill your hole.

1 large sweet potato, peeled and
    cut into ½cm (¼ inch) slices
2 large red onions, finely sliced
as much cheese as you dare,
    but we put 100g (3½oz/1 cup)
    extra mature Cheddar in ours
3 thick slices of ham
3 large eggs, plus the whites from
    4 more eggs
125ml (4 fl oz/½ cup) milk
a pinch of mustard powder
a pinch of salt
lots of freshly ground black
    pepper

You'll need a decent 23cm (9 inch) deep dish – silicone is always easier as you can just tip the quiche straight out.

Preheat the oven to 180°C fan/400°F/gas mark 6.

Spray your dish with a little spray oil and layer in the sliced sweet potato, making sure to cover the bottom entirely and some of the sides if you can – don't fret if it's uneven, it'll soften down and smarten up under the weight of the quiche filling. Pop it into the oven for 25 minutes or so.

Sweat the onions in a pan with a splash of oil until softened.

Grate your cheese and cut the ham into small cubes.

Mix the eggs, egg whites, milk, mustard powder, salt and pepper together in a jug.

Take your sweet potatoes out of the oven and gently tidy up the layer to make sure there are no holes. Cover the sweet potatoes with the cheese, ham and onions, then top with the egg mixture.

Cook in the oven for about 35 minutes. If it looks as though it is burning, cover the top with foil. The quiche is done when it's still a wee bit wobbly but a knife pushed into the middle comes out clean. Leave to cool – it'll firm up nicely.

Serve with salad to the delight of your waiting audience.

Note from Paul
This freezes superbly and is perfect for lunch the next day.

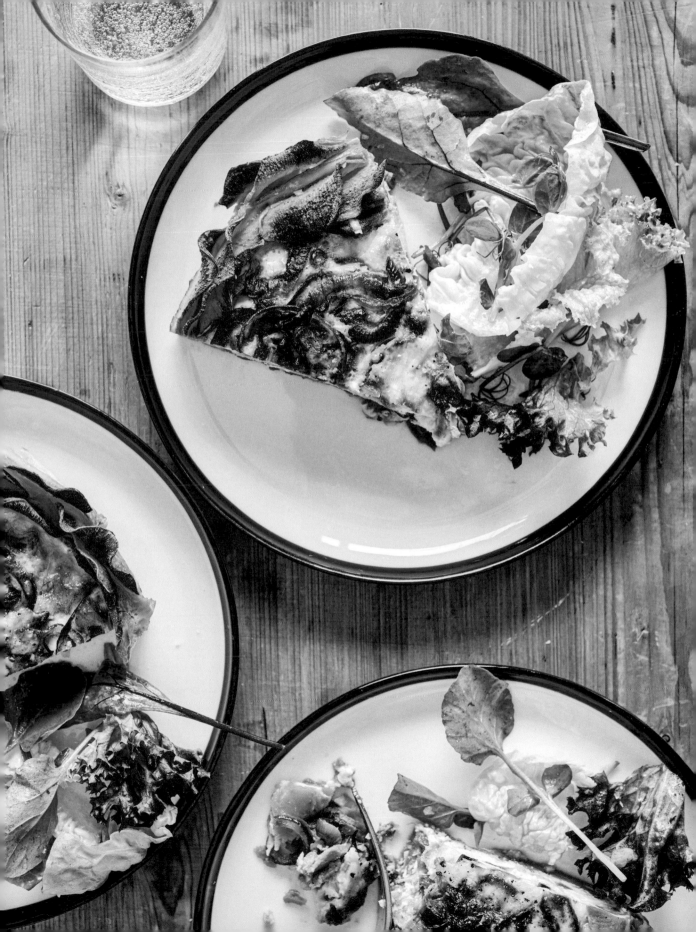

● ● ● ● ● ●

IN-&-OUT WRAPS

Serves 1

Each without any fillings:

270 calories for red

238 calories for green

235 calories for orange

1 or 2 eggs
a pinch of black pepper and salt

For '**red**' ham and tomato wraps, blitz in a handful of ham and the flesh (but not the seeds) from a couple of tomatoes.

For '**green**' spinach and feta wraps, a handful of fresh spinach leaves and a few cubes of feta.

For '**orange**' spicy pepper wraps, half a small orange pepper, diced, and a pinch of chilli flakes.

Any leftover peppers, tomatoes, spinach, etc. can all go inside the wrap once cooked

We're calling these in-and-out wraps because they've got goodness mixed inside the wraps and outside.

They came about entirely by accident when we were reminiscing about the time we tried to make a slimming roulade. Back in the days when we were naive and thought a kilo of sweetener was enough to make something palatable. What we ended up eating both looked and tasted like a well-worn dishcloth stuffed with strawberries. You'll see that we make up for this later in the book.

These are great to make in the morning and wrap up for lunch, though we would advise against adding 'wet' fillings if you're keeping them sweating in your bag until noon. They work best if you have a proper blender (just for speed) but, failing that, a stick blender whacked into a jug will do just fine. Simply make up your wrap and stuff it with whatever colourful trappings you have rattling around in the fridge.

We tend to use two eggs per wrap because it makes it more substantial, but if you're wanting a few, just drop it down to one egg. It'll be thinner and more delicate, but then so are we. For this recipe, it's very much an add-what-you-like affair, so we've simply given you three options for wraps and fillings – but do feel free to swap them out.

Crack the egg into a blender with the salt and pepper, then add your 'mix-ins' and whiz – you don't want it blended to a paste, but rather just mixed together so there's still a bit of 'chunkiness' to it.

Spray a small non-stick frying pan with oil and pop it over a medium heat. Tip your egg mixture into the pan and allow it to settle. Cook it like a pancake – when it's set and reasonably firm, throw caution to the wind and flip.

Cook it for a moment more, then slide it out on to a plate – it'll be easier to fold while warm.

Fill with whatever you like, following the instructions shown below, then cut horizontally on the diagonal for that fresh, meal-deal look.

For filling ideas, we like to use anything we happen across in the fridge – jarred cooked peppers, mushrooms, sun-dried tomatoes, cold meats, soft cheese, houmous, refried beans, smoked cheese, salad leaves, cottage cheese – the list is endless, though don't be a scamp and add pork pies. Hard to fold!

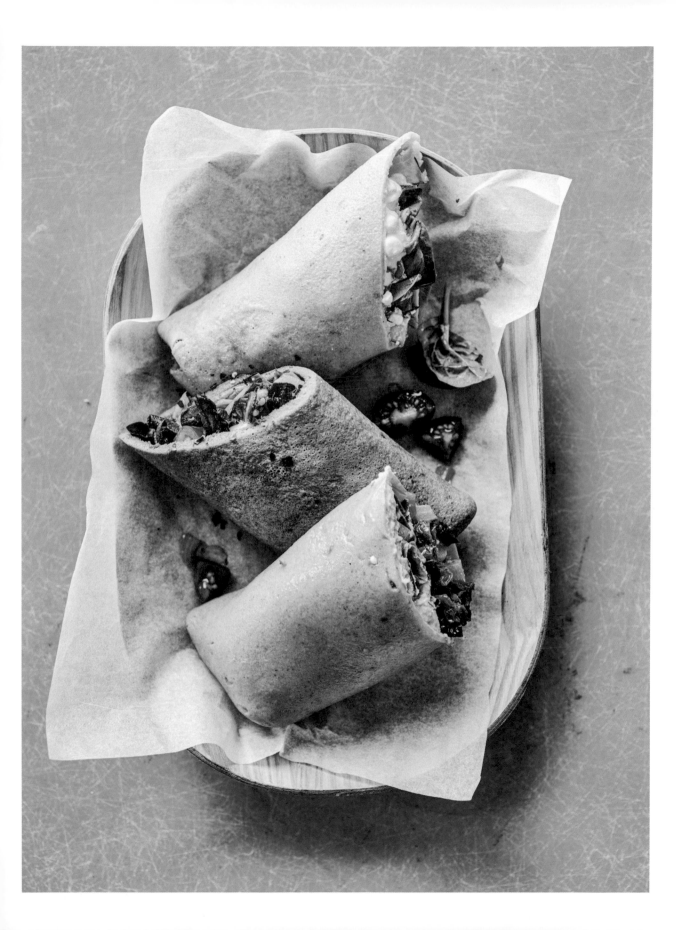

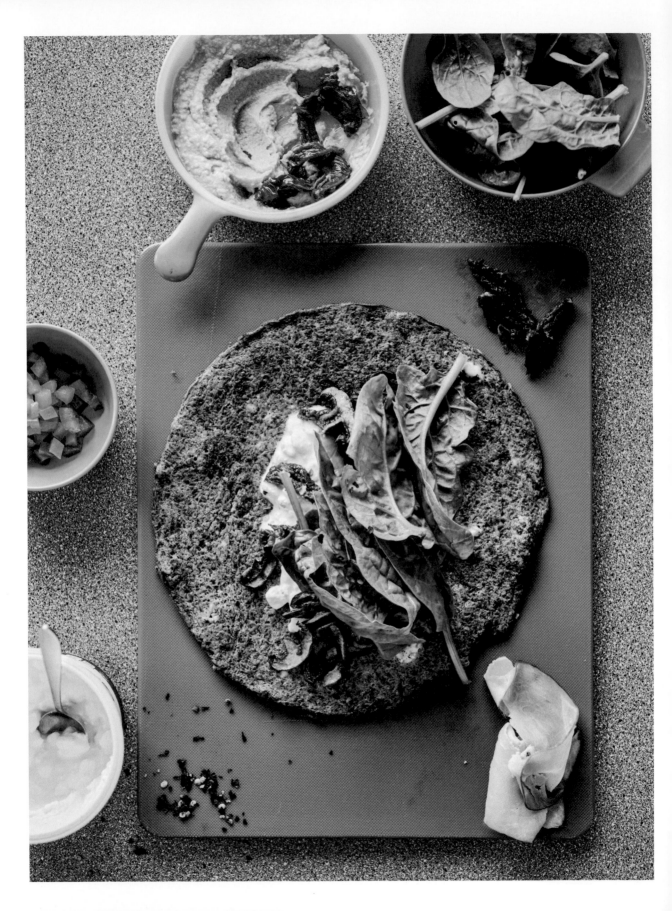

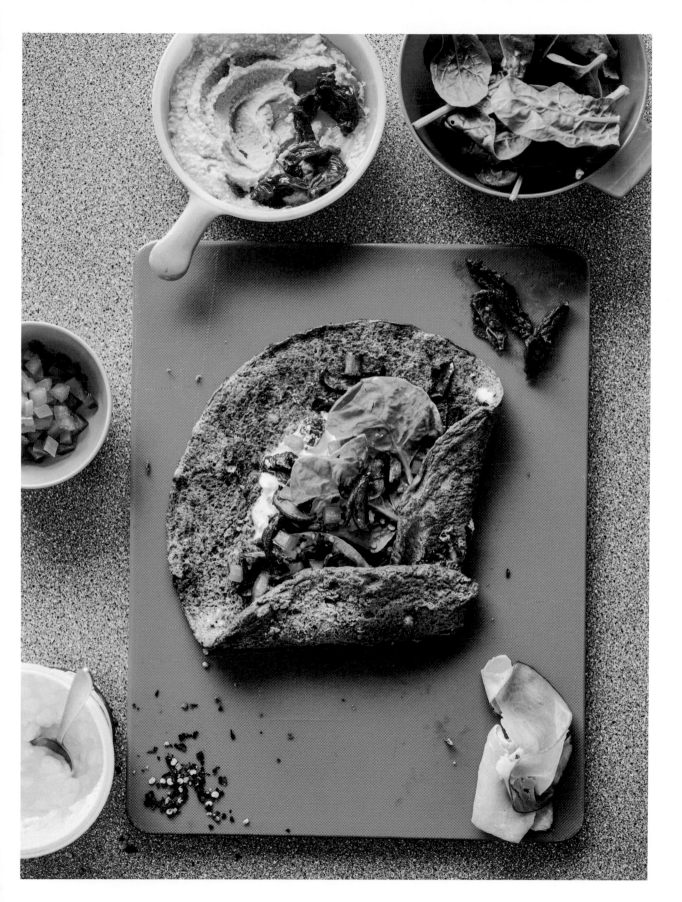

● ● ● ● ● ●

HEALTHY HOUMOUS

Makes a big bowlful

For a 50g (1¾oz) serving:

52 calories for lemon and garlic

62 calories for parmesan and basil

68 calories for paprika and sun-dried tomato

51 calories for pickled red cabbage dip

1 × 400g (14oz) tin of chickpeas, drained and rinsed
2 large tablespoons cottage cheese
1 clove of garlic, peeled
a pinch of sea salt
1 tablespoon lemon juice

Houmous is one of my victories over Paul – he spent years pulling a face like a cat's bum at the thought of it. His idea of a 'posh dip' was one of those four-way dips you get in the fridge aisle at the supermarket, which might as well come with half a broken breadstick in them to save time. I would try to open his mind to fancy dipping appurtenances but he would have none of it. We had arguments a-plenty where we would tussle over taramasalata, square off over salsa and get the hump over houmous. (You may wonder – we do indeed theme all our domestics around alliterative verbs. It keeps things spicy.) I finally won Paul over by tricking him into thinking it was an especially gritty white chocolate dip. The fact that he paired that with a barbecue Pringle should tell you everything you need to know about him.

I'm sure it's an abomination to call this houmous, given the omission of olive oil and tahini, the two key components of a delicious houmous. But I care not: it tastes amazing, is the perfect carrier for all sorts of flavours, and frankly, if you don't enjoy dipping your cucumber in this, then you're dead inside. To help you, we've included four spins on the basic recipe to keep you entertained.

Blend all the ingredients together in a blitzer, adjusting the amounts slightly depending on how thick and chunky you like your houmous.

For lemon and garlic, add a couple of extra garlic cloves, a dash more lemon juice and some very finely grated lemon peel, being careful not to take the pith.

For basil and Parmesan, add 15 fresh basil leaves and 20g (¾oz/¼ cup) of grated Parmesan together with a pinch of salt.

For paprika and sun-dried tomato, add a few sun-dried tomatoes together with a little of the oil they came in, and decorate with a pinch of sweet paprika.

For a pickled red cabbage dip, just add some – shock horror – pickled red cabbage together with a dash of the pickling vinegar it came in.

Note from Paul
This is very much a 'make on the day' recipe, as it doesn't freeze especially well – but as it only takes less than a minute to throw together, that shouldn't pose a difficulty.

WE LIKE TO CHOP A SELECTION OF DIFFERENT VEGETABLES INTO STICKS, PRESENT THEM ATTRACTIVELY ON A PLATE, THEN IGNORE THEM ENTIRELY WHILE WE EAT CRISPS.

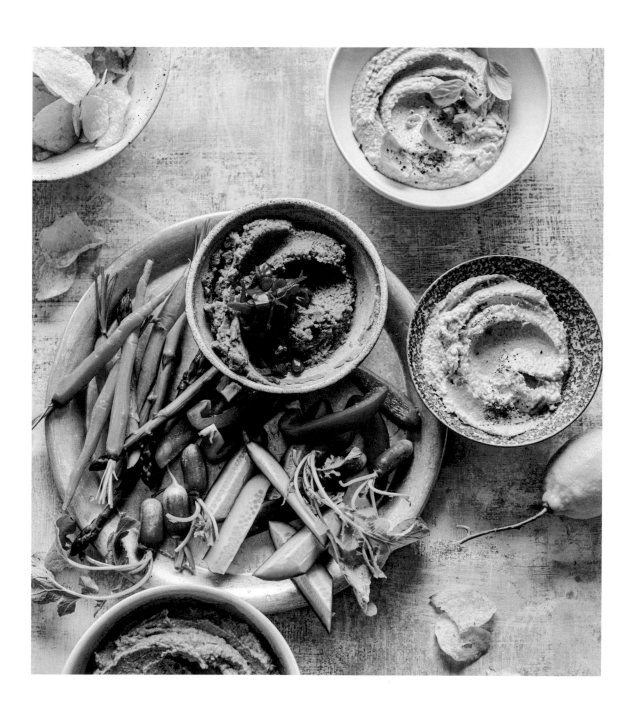

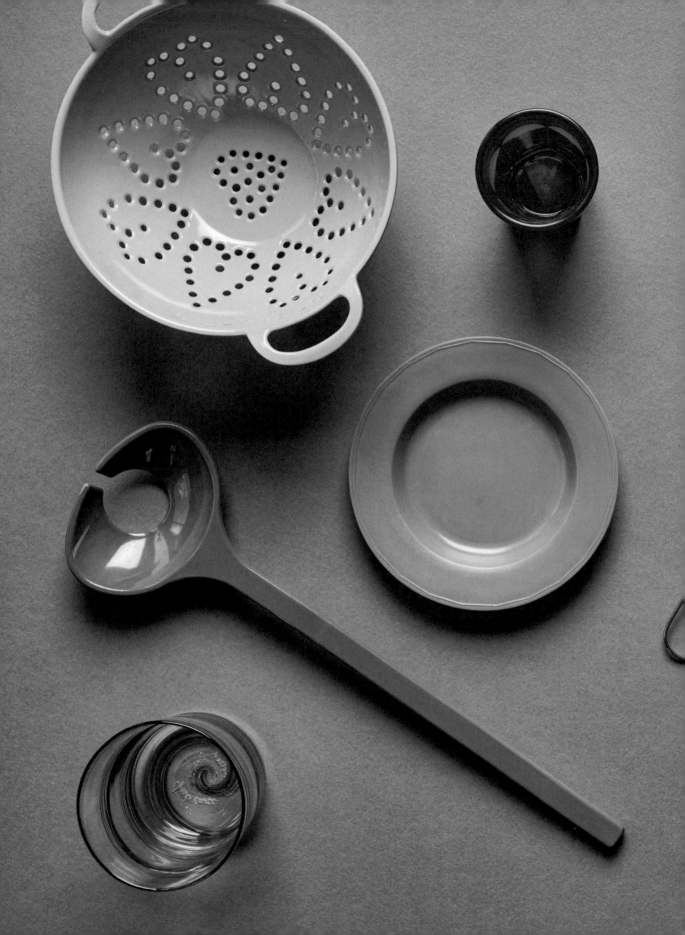

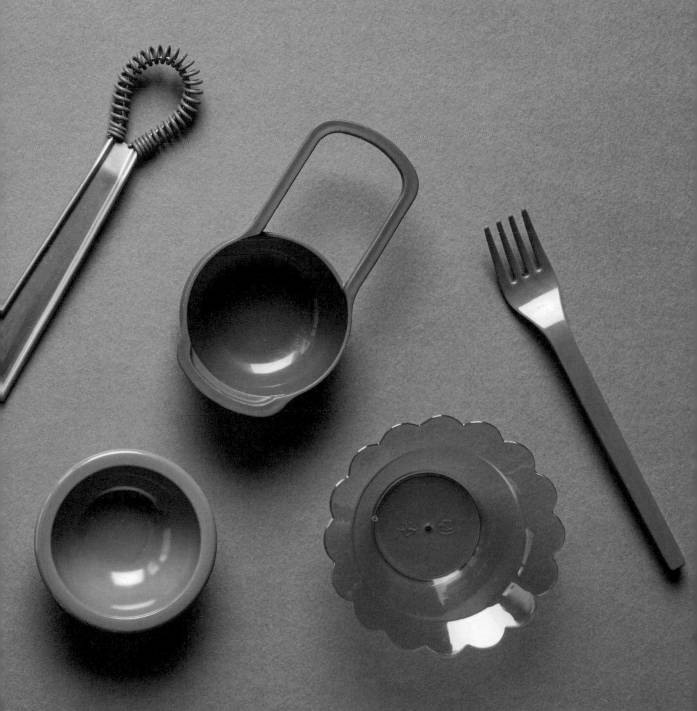

MEAT-FREE MARVELS

● ● ● ● ● ●

ROASTED RAINBOW CARBONARA

Serves 4
468 calories

This is a two-part recipe, in that you'll need to roast your veg first before making it into a carbonara, but if you're savvy like us you'll do a massive tray of vegetables and keep some aside in the fridge – they're perfect for chucking into salads, couscous or wraps. The carbonara side of things takes no time at all, so don't fret.

This makes enough for two massive bowls of deliciousness, with lots of leftover vegetables. We've used vegetables that make for a colourful plate, but honestly, anything you have cluttering the bottom of the fridge will do just fine.

Top tip though: cut all your vegetables to almost the same size. You can season the vegetables with any different seasonings you may have kicking about, but we're all about simplicity here at Chubby Towers.

1 egg, plus the yolks from 4 more
60g (2¼oz/¾ cup) grated
    Parmesan cheese
200g (7oz) dried spaghetti
a handful of fresh peas

For the roasted veg
1 large orange pepper, cut into
    small chunks
1 courgette, cut into chunks
1 large red onion, cut into chunks
1 small head of broccoli, cut into
    small trees
250g (9oz) mix of yellow and
    red cherry tomatoes, halved
    (keep aside from the rest of
    the vegetables to begin with)
2 tablespoons of olive oil
    (or a few sprays of low-fat
    cooking spray, if you prefer)
a pinch or 2 of coarse salt and
    freshly ground black pepper

Preheat your oven to 170°C fan/375°F/gas mark 5 and find a good non-stick roasting tray.

Put your vegetables into a bowl (everything bar the tomatoes and the peas, that is), then drizzle over the oil, sprinkle with salt and pepper and give everything a good shake around. Arrange the vegetables on the tray and bake for 15 minutes.

In the same oily bowl you used for the first batch of veg, throw the tomatoes around so they get coated and a little bit bashed.

Once the 15 minutes are up, give everything a turn and add the tomatoes. Cook for another 10 minutes before checking that everything has softened a little – a bit of crunch is fine.

While the veg are cooking, beat the egg with the 4 yolks, adding most of the Parmesan and a generous amount of black pepper, and set aside.

When the vegetables are ready, pop your spaghetti on, cook it according to the packet instructions, then drain, keeping aside a cup of the starchy cooking water, and return the spaghetti to the pan.

Pour the egg mixture through the spaghetti and mix well – make sure the spaghetti is still hot when you do this so the sauce cooks. Add a little of the reserved cooking water if you need to.

Tip in the peas and as much of the roasted vegetables as you like, and serve topped with more Parmesan.

Notes from Paul
- *You can add meat if you like – lardons, ham and shredded chicken all go well in this recipe, but we like to have a meat-free day.*
- *You can roast whole garlic cloves alongside the vegetables. Roasted garlic is a joy, but you'll need to pack some Polos for after.*

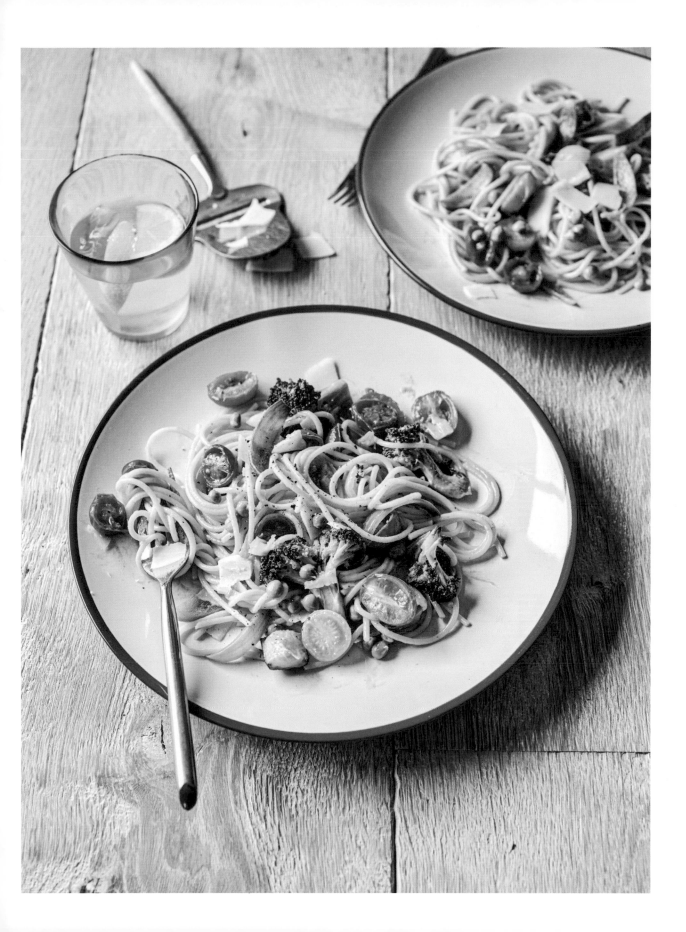

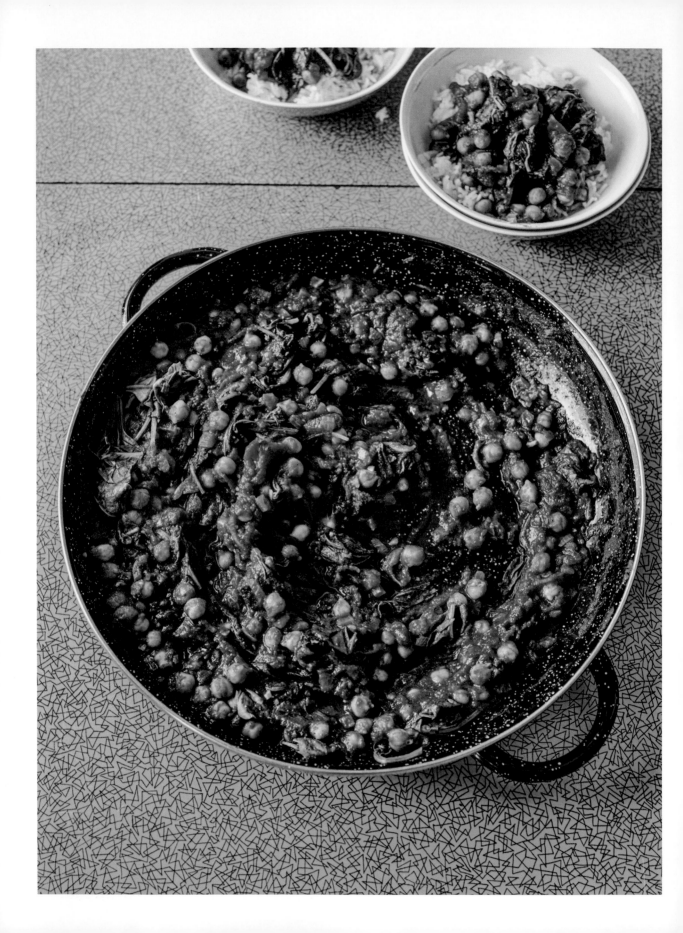

TOMATO & CHICKPEA STEW

Serves 4
154 calories

1 red onion, finely chopped
3 cloves of garlic, minced
1 tablespoon tomato purée
2 teaspoons ground cumin
1 teaspoon paprika
½ teaspoon hot chilli powder
2 × 400g (14oz) tins of tomatoes
½ teaspoon salt
½ teaspoon freshly ground black
   pepper
2 teaspoons honey
1 × 400g (14oz) tin of chickpeas,
   drained and rinsed
200g (7oz) baby spinach

This recipe came about thanks to one of a few wonderful sets of neighbours that we have, who I'll namecheck just to make sure they keep looking after the cats when we go off on our jaunts. I jest, they're truly lovely folks: Wilf and Wilma.

When we moved here, they took us under their wing and became the perfect neighbours: chatty without being nosy, friendly without inviting themselves round for sugar and gossip. One of the perks of having our excellent neighbours is that barely a week goes by in the summer without a surfeit of vegetables being handed over from their allotment. Some weeks it's enough aubergines to make a convent blush, other times it's eighty-seven leeks and a wheelbarrow of turnips. This recipe stems from a glut of tomatoes that he left on my doorstep. I mean, I love tomatoes, and heartily encourage you as a reader to set away a little cherry tomato plant at your earliest opportunity because nothing beats home-grown tomatoes, but there's only so many things you can do with them.

Mind, I'll take bags of vegetables any time over the game birds he sometimes leaves hanging from my front door handle. It was four weeks into our new home when I came back from work to find a dead pheasant on my doormat. He's lucky I didn't report it as a hate crime, frankly.

Now, you'll see that we have used tinned tomatoes in this recipe rather than fresh – that's because we wanted a 'quick' take on our recipe. If you have the time, about 500g (1lb or so) of fresh, skinned cherry tomatoes will make this dish sing. When I say fresh, mind, I mean it. Greenhouse or bust.

Heat a large frying pan over a medium-high heat and spray with a little oil. Add the onions and gently cook until they start to go translucent, then add the garlic and stir well for a minute or 2.

Add the tomato purée, cumin, paprika and chilli powder, and stir well.

Add the tinned tomatoes and gently crush with a wooden spoon as you stir them. Add the salt, pepper and honey and simmer over a low heat until thickened.

Add the drained chickpeas to the pan and stir through to warm them up.

Add the spinach and stir in well until wilted, then serve.

Note from Paul
This tastes great served with rice.

CREAMY GARLIC MUSHROOMS ON CHEESY FRIED POLENTA

Serves 4
318 calories

1 litre (1¾ pints/4 cups) good
    vegetable stock
180g (6½oz/1 cup) polenta
    (see notes below)
50g (1¾oz/½ cup) reduced-fat
    Cheddar cheese, grated
    (optional)
200g (7oz/3 cups) wild
    mushrooms
2 cloves of garlic, crushed
3 tablespoons crème fraîche
    (though see notes below
    for a cheat)
a couple of good handfuls
    of watercress
salt and pepper

It has taken years to win Paul around to mushrooms – he was always one of those folks who turned their nose up at the thought of them. I thought he was being a fussy little boob, as per his usual stance. However, digging a little deeper, it turns out his mycological ire stems from his first job, which happened to be on a local mushroom farm.

At the tender age of sixteen, his sole duty was to walk up rows upon rows of growing mushrooms and moisten the fertilizer – a potent mix of fine soil and chicken manure – with warm water. Something about spending your teenage years cloaked in a miasma of chicken effluence didn't appeal and so he nicked off after sticking it out for two days.

Bring your stock to the boil in a pan, then lower the heat to a medium simmer. Start adding your polenta – apologies, but it's going to take a long while of stirring, adding more polenta and stirring again – you want this thick and able to hold itself (just like I wish my husband could). Once the polenta is close to being just right, add a good few pinches of salt and pepper along with the cheese, if using, then stir again. For the want of a better term, slop the polenta out into a baking tray lined with greaseproof paper and make it as even as possible – it doesn't need to fill the tray, but it should be about 1.5cm (about ¾ inch) thick. Chill in the fridge for an hour or so.

When you're ready for the next part, roughly chop your mushrooms. Spray the bottom of a good non-stick frying pan with a little oil and gently fry your crushed garlic, then tumble in the mushrooms. Cook them for about 10 minutes, until they have reduced and softened, then remove with a slotted spoon and place in a separate pan (keeping the oily frying pan for later). Stir through the crème fraîche and leave on the lowest possible heat just to keep warm.

Take your cooled polenta and, using a circular cookie cutter (or a knife if you're handy), cut yourself some 'cakes' or slabs of polenta. Heat your oiled pan again over a medium heat, adding a few more sprays of olive oil. Using a fish slice, carefully place your polenta in the pan. Fry for around 2–3 minutes, until brown, then carefully flip the pieces over.

To serve, stack the polenta cakes at the bottom of a dish, layer on some watercress and top with the cheesy garlic mushrooms.

Notes from Paul
- *You can speed this recipe up by using ready-made polenta, which is sold in blocks and is perfect for slicing, frying and serving up. However, it's also much higher in calories. Fair warning.*
- *If you can't be fussed to make the creamy sauce, simply whack some garlic and herb cream cheese through your mushrooms.*

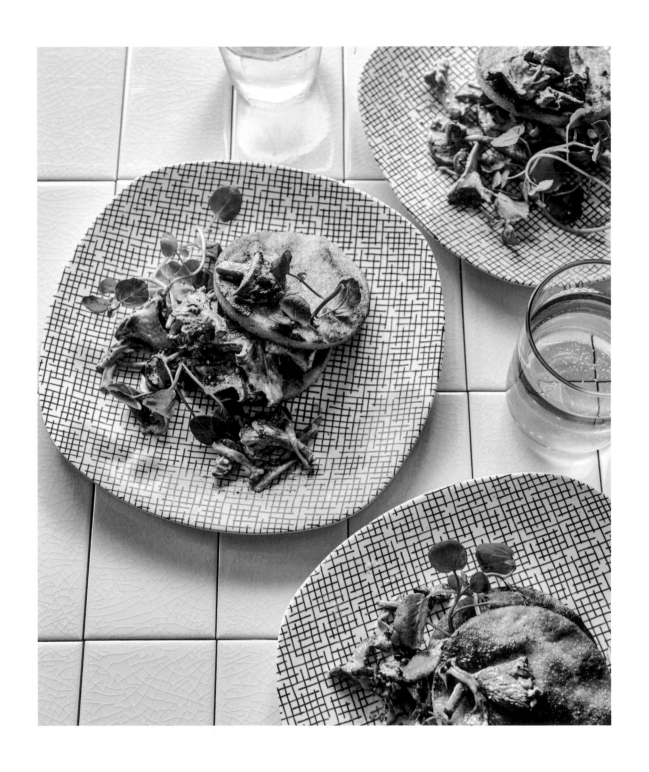

DO NOT FRET IF THE POLENTA FALLS APART;
YOU'RE EATING IT, NOT TURNING IT INTO AN
ART INSTALLATION.

● ● ● ● ● ●

THREE-BEAN COWBOY STEW

Serves 6
422 calories

1 large red pepper, finely diced
1 large white onion, finely diced
1 small red chilli, chopped, if you
 like it spicy
3 cloves of garlic, crushed
1 tablespoon hot chilli powder
1 teaspoon smoked paprika
1 teaspoon ground cumin
1 × 400g (14oz) tin of chopped
 tomatoes
1 × 400g (14oz) tin of baked
 beans (use BBQ beans if you
 can find them)
1 × 400g (14oz) tin of butter
 beans, drained and rinsed
1 × 400g (14oz) tin of red kidney
 beans, drained and rinsed
1 large sweet potato, peeled
 and cut into chunks
300g (10½oz/1½ cups) red lentils
8 sun-dried tomatoes (see note)
1 tablespoon Worcestershire
 sauce
1 litre (1¾ pints/4 cups) stock –
 we use beef stock but if you
 want to keep it veggie, swap it
 out for a vegetarian alternative

Cowboy stew has been doing the rounds for years – a large chunk of gammon slow-cooked with beans and served shredded over rice (there's a fantastic recipe on our blog, just sayin'), but sometimes it's nice to put the meat away. It looks like there's a lot of ingredients but it's mostly tins – this is a recipe that takes no time to prepare and will do all the work for you while burbling away on the hob.

Like all stews, the longer you leave it the better it tastes – so make sure you keep some aside for a jacket potato topping the next day.

Find a decent pan that will hold all your ingredients.

Gently fry the red pepper, onion and chilli in a little oil, adding the crushed garlic, chilli powder, smoked paprika and cumin for a couple of minutes at the end.

Tip everything else into the pan and give it all a good stir. Bring to the boil, then leave to simmer over a low heat for an hour or 2 – do keep checking on it lest it needs a touch more stock.

When you're ready to serve, ladle it out over cooked rice and deliver with a smile.

Notes from Paul
- *We like to use dehydrated sun-dried tomatoes rather than those in oil – they take about 10 minutes to hydrate in boiling water and you can keep the water to add to the stew.*
- *Chopped tomatoes with chilli and BBQ beans will add to the flavours but aren't essential.*

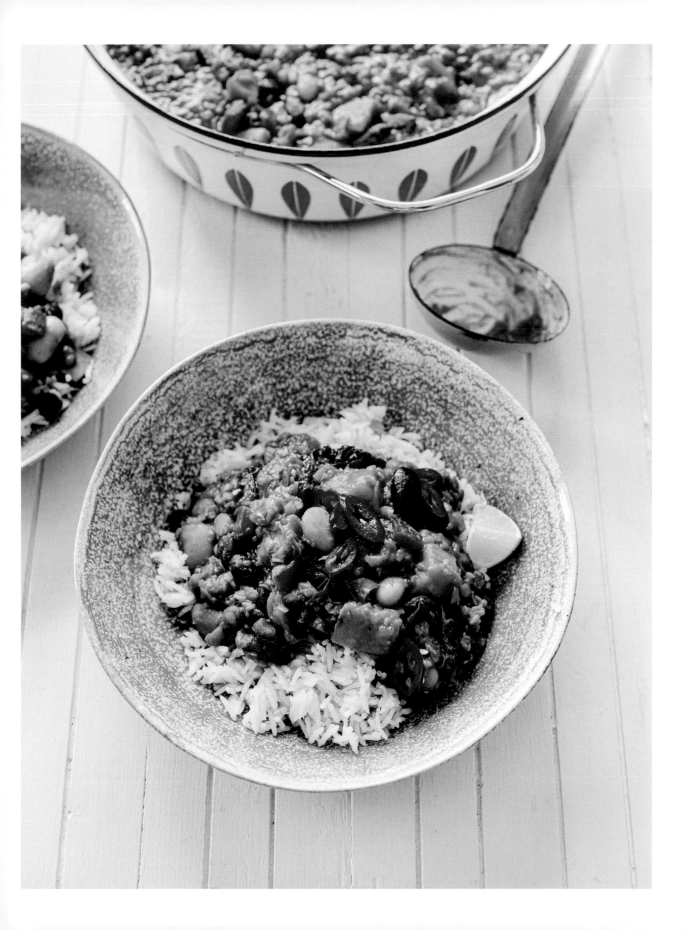

STUFFED SPINACH & RICOTTA CANNELLONI

Serves 4
499 calories

1 small red onion, finely chopped
1 clove of garlic, crushed
½ teaspoon fennel seeds
2 × 400g (14oz) tins of chopped
    tomatoes
a pinch of sugar (optional)
18 cannelloni tubes (buy 24 –
    there's always a few breaks)
500g (1lb 2oz) fresh spinach
250g (8¾oz/1 cup) ricotta
200g (7oz/1 cup) reduced-fat
    cottage cheese, drained,
    so the curds remain
75g (2¾oz/¾ cup) reduced-fat
    mature Cheddar cheese,
    grated
a pinch of nutmeg
1 egg
fresh basil leaves, to adorn the
    top, and as much extra cheese
    as you could possibly want

When I told Paul I was going to include the stuffed cannelloni recipe, he seemed downcast. I asked him: Paul, a penne for your thoughts? The silly bugger thought I'd stuff the intro with a fusilli pasta puns! We argued and he went to bed, cross, leaving me cannelloni. I knew I couldn't get away with it – orzo it seemed … But then, bigoli, inspiration struck! I'd do it anyway! Least I wasn't dishing up alphabetti spaghetti – that could have spelled disaster.*

To start, make the tomato sauce by gently frying the onion, garlic and fennel seeds in a pan over a medium heat. Pour the tomatoes into the pan and allow to gently bubble, adding a pinch of sugar only if you think it tastes a bit acidic – leave it cooking while you fill the tubes.

In another pan – as big as you can – boil enough water to allow the cannelloni tubes to gently bob around for a minute or so – you want to soften them, not cook them through. It can be easier to do these a few at a time so they don't stick together. Remove with a slotted spoon and leave to cool while you prepare the filling.

Preheat the oven to 180°C fan/400°F/gas mark 6.

Pour out all but a dribble of the water you used for the pasta (enough so the bottom of the pan is just covered) and add your spinach to the pan. Give it a few stirs until it has wilted down, then drain. You want to remove as much moisture as you can here – we pile the spinach on to one chopping board, place another over the top, then squeeze like a sandwich – when you think you've finished, squeeze again!

Finely chop your spinach and tip it into a mixing bowl with the ricotta, cottage cheese curds, mature Cheddar, nutmeg and egg – stir everything together until really well mixed.

Now the tricky part – spoon the mixture into the tubes, or, if you're clumsy and cack-handed like us, fill a large sandwich bag with half the mixture, cut off a corner, and you have an easy piping bag. Squeeze gently, filling the cannelloni at both ends.

Once they're all done – and don't worry, there will be breakages, but you can use them to fill any gaps in the dish – spread a few spoonfuls of the tomato sauce across the bottom of an overproof dish, then layer the cannelloni side by side and top to top in an orderly fashion.

Pour over the remainder of the sauce, cover with foil, and pop the dish into the oven for around 25 minutes. Take it out and top with more cheese, then put it under the grill for around 10 minutes, until golden.

Garnish with the basil leaves and serve with a simple salad, or chips if you're feeling outrageously carby.

* The Twochubbycubs would like to unreservedly apologise to our readers for the tortured puns in the intro just now. We knew what we were doing and did it anyway – we have no excuses for the splits in your side or the wheezing you have from laughing yourself silly.

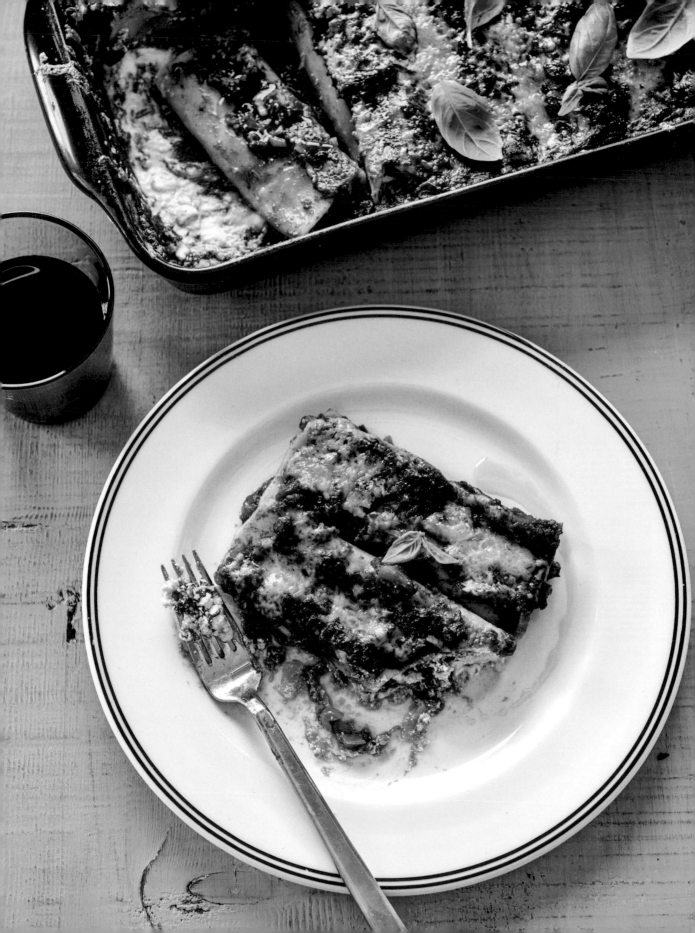

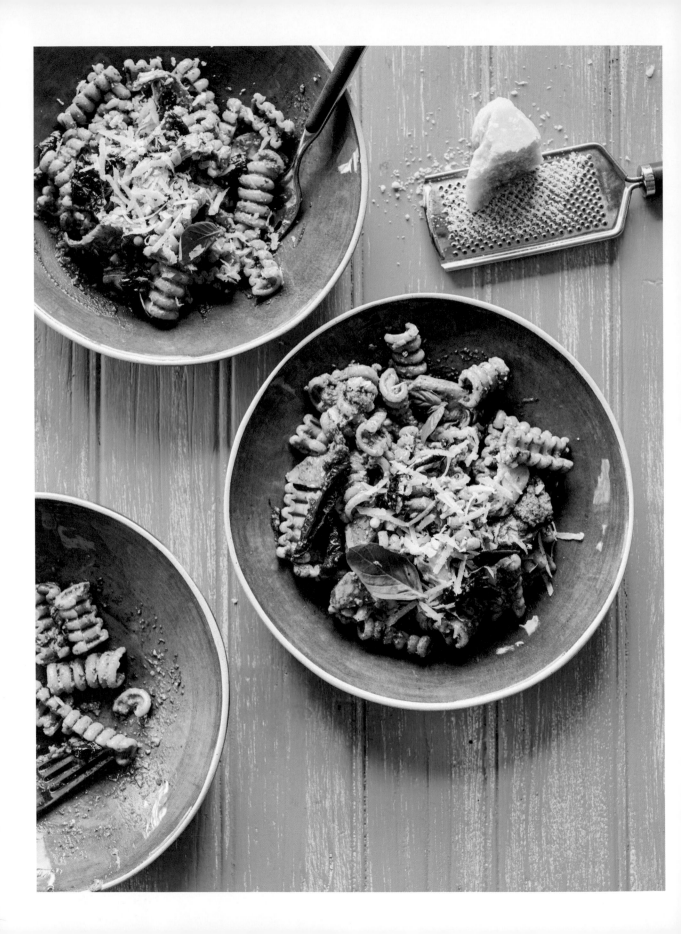

PESTO & GOAT'S CHEESE PASTA

Serves 4
366 calories

You have ITV to thank for this recipe – we were given a plateful of it to eat backstage while waiting to go on our 'LOOK HOW FAT WE ARE' segment on This Time Next Year. I think they secretly wanted us to look as bloated as possible before filming, though they needn't have bothered: we came bouncing through that door like someone trying to squeeze a party balloon through a letterbox. However, it stuck with us and we've managed to make an excellent approximation of it at home.

That was a joy, mind, having so many people fuss over us in a vain attempt to make us look halfway presentable in high-definition. You have to understand that Paul and I are absolute minimalists when it comes to a beauty regime – cold splash of water in the evening before bed, hot shower in the morning and a bar of coal-tar soap. It's like living in prison. The only reason I haven't grown my hair back is because it is altogether too much effort to maintain. At least this way I can shave my head and claim it's because I like the mean'n'moody snooker ball look.

250g (9oz/2½ cups) dried pasta

50g (1¾oz/¼ cup) soft goat's cheese

125g (4½oz/⅔ cup) reduced-fat green pesto

160g (5½oz) tinned artichoke hearts, drained and chopped

30g (1oz) sun-dried tomatoes, chopped

2 tablespoons grated Parmesan cheese, to serve

Cook the pasta according to the packet instructions, then drain (reserving some of the pasta water in a mug).

While the pasta is cooking, mix together the goat's cheese and pesto in a bowl.

When the pasta is cooked and drained, tip it into the pesto bowl and stir until well mixed – add a tablespoon of the reserved pasta water at a time to loosen it if needed.

Add the artichokes and tomatoes and stir again until well combined, then serve, sprinkled with the Parmesan.

Notes from Paul

· *Use whatever pasta you have lying around in your cupboards – anything will do!*

· *This is also delicious with some shredded chicken breast mixed in, if you fancy a bit of meat.*

· *To save on the calories, look for the sun-dried tomatoes that aren't in oil – they'll need a bit of plumping in hot water first, but they'll taste just as good.*

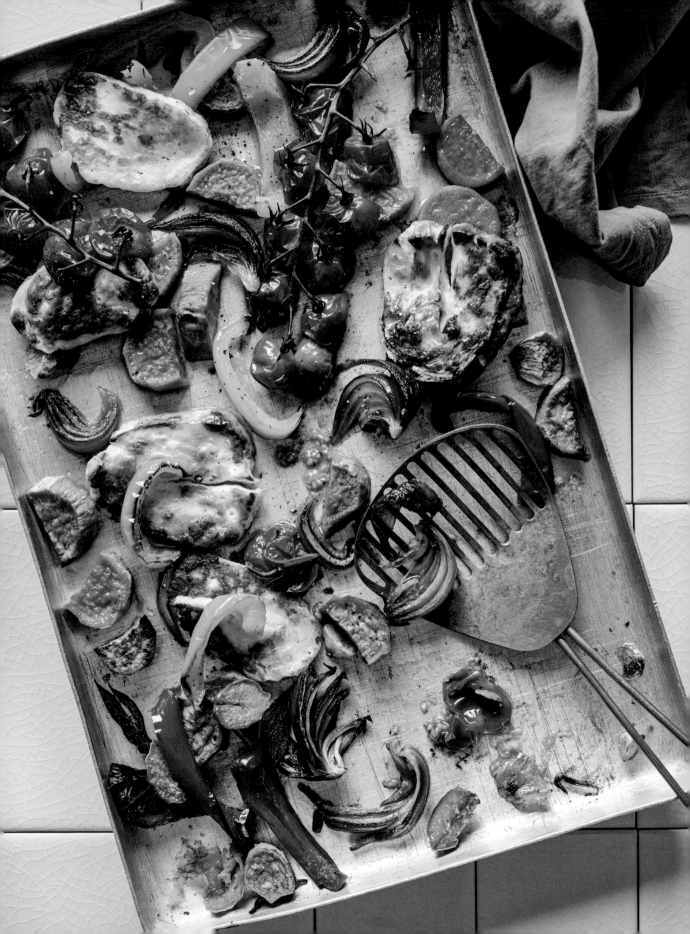

● ● ○ ● ● ●

SWEET POTATO
& HALLOUMI BAKE

Serves 4
238 calories

A sweet potato and halloumi bake – no, hear us out, it might not strike you as a substantial dish and indeed, we'd class it more as a light lunch, but damn it's a good one. Reminds me of my dad for two reasons – sweet potatoes are about the one vegetable he'd never managed to grow, and plus, halloumi sounds like a Geordie person shouting down the platform from a departing train. My dad, much to Paul's eternal aural consternation, is proper Geordie.

My dad is brilliant, and I don't tell him often enough, so where better place than in his own son's book? I'm everything my dad isn't: cack-handed when it comes to DIY, clueless around the garden, flamboyantly homosexual.

He never raises an eyebrow when I ring up shrieking because I need a shelf putting up or a lightbulb has gone out and, between Paul's weight and my dizziness, we can't get up on a ladder to change it. For that he is a hero. I'd invite him round for dinner but if I served him this, he'd sweep it away, pronounce it veggie muck and put his own bacon on. Champion.

For the record, Paul's dad – and his lovely wife, Wendy – are both absolute treasures.

400g (14oz) sweet potatoes, peeled and cut into 4cm (1½ inch) chunks
1 red pepper, sliced
1 yellow pepper, sliced
1 onion, cut into wedges
a good handful of cherry tomatoes
6 cloves of garlic, finely chopped
125g (4½ oz) halloumi, sliced

Preheat the oven to 180°C fan/400°F/gas mark 6.

Put the sweet potatoes, peppers, onion, tomatoes and garlic into a large bowl and spray with oil. Gently tumble, spraying with oil a few times to ensure everything is well coated.

Spread the vegetables out on to a large baking sheet and roast in the oven for 45 minutes.

Place the halloumi under a medium-high grill for 5 minutes, then combine with the roasted vegetables before serving.

• • • • • •

VEGETARIAN MOUSSAKA

Serves 4
393 calories

Moussaka was one of the very first dishes we made when we joined up to slimming classes so many moons ago. I spent an age chopping vegetables, making the sauce, measuring out our cheese allowance and layering everything just so. I must have been trying to get into Paul's knickers at the time because now everything is prepared with all the care and attention of someone trying to escape a house fire.

Anyway, when it was ready to come out of the oven, I walked into the kitchen, lifted the dish out proudly and turned to show Paul, only for the dish to shatter in my hands. Naturally, with my touch for the theatrical, I assumed I'd been shot through the kitchen window and threw myself shrieking to the floor, landing boob-down on a scalding slice of aubergine. This induced more screaming, of course, and well, there was no way back from that – I believe we spent the night navigating a Chinese takeaway while I rubbed Savlon into my nipple.

So yes: moussaka. Mind how you take it out of the oven, won't you?

1 onion, diced
2 × 400g (14oz) tins of chopped
    tomatoes
2 teaspoons dried mixed herbs
1 bay leaf
3 large aubergines
800g (1lb 12oz) potatoes, cut into
    5mm (¼ inch) slices
200g (7oz/1 cup) extra-light soft
    cheese
1 egg
a pinch of ground cinnamon
2 large courgettes, sliced thinly
100g (3½oz/¾ cup) reduced-fat
    feta cheese, crumbled

Place a large frying pan over a medium heat and spray with a little oil.

Add the onion and cook for 4–5 minutes, stirring frequently.

Add the tomatoes, mixed herbs and bay leaf and stir well, then reduce the heat and simmer for 25–30 minutes, stirring occasionally.

Preheat the oven to 180°C fan/400°F/gas mark 6.

Cut the tops off the aubergines and cut them lengthways into 5mm (¼ inch) slices. Spray both sides of the slices with oil and place under a hot grill for 3–4 minutes on each side, then remove and set aside.

Bring a large pan of salted water to the boil. Add the sliced potatoes and simmer for 4–5 minutes, then carefully drain.

Mix the soft cheese, egg and cinnamon together in a bowl and set aside.

Spoon a layer of the tomato sauce into the bottom of a large baking dish. Spread over half the aubergine slices, half the courgette slices and follow with half the potatoes.

Spoon over half the remaining tomato sauce, followed by the rest of the aubergines and potatoes, and spoon the remaining sauce on top.

Carefully spread the soft cheese mixture over the top and crumble over the feta.

Bake in the oven for 1 hour, or until everything is softened and the top is browned.

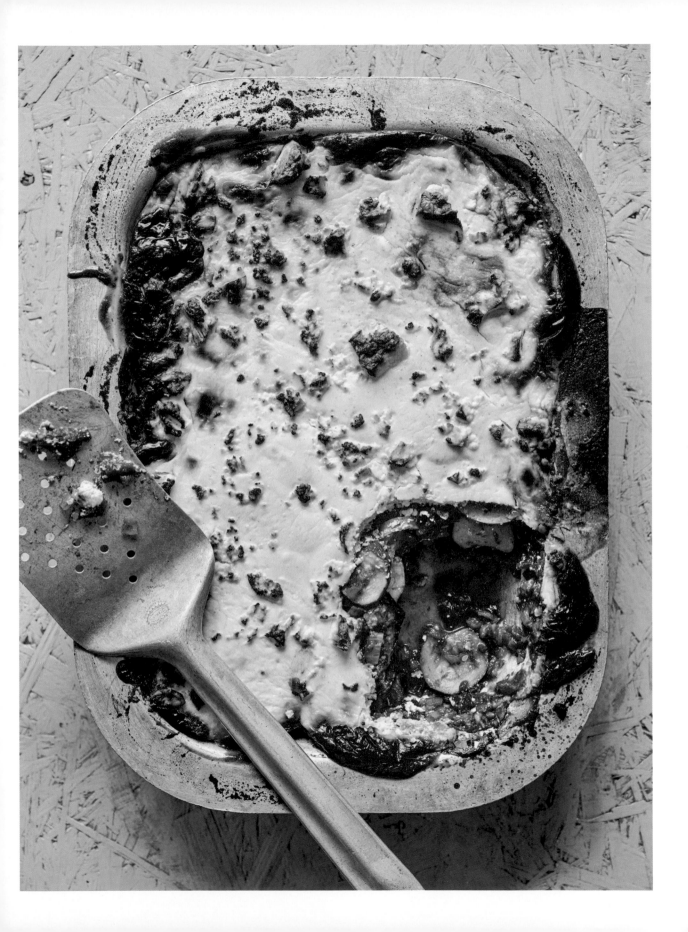

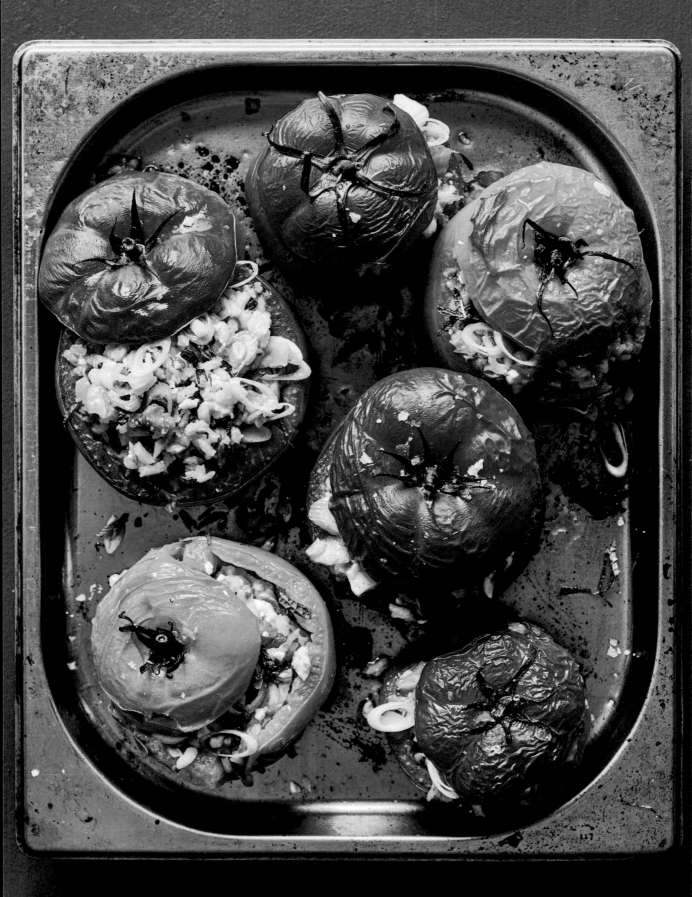

TOMATOES STUFFED WITH RICE

Serves 4
165 calories

100g (3½oz/½ cup) Arborio rice
4 large beefsteak tomatoes
a handful of fresh mint
100g (3½oz/¾ cup) reduced-fat
    feta cheese, crumbled
3 fat spring onions, sliced as thin
    as you dare
2 cloves of garlic, crushed

This dish has been rattling around in my recipe bank for years – it even predates Paul, and certainly predates my respect for him. I used to knock about with a charming lady who doubled as my flatmate for a good year. She was what one might call a casual vegetarian, in that she would have excellent ideas of saving the planet and never having anything die for her dinner until she was absolutely steaming and fancied a dirty kebab. This recipe was one of hers and a favourite of mine – she would present me with a plate of these to try to soften me every time she had missed her rent payment. Ah, good times.

Cook your rice according to the packet instructions and set aside.

Preheat the oven to 180°C fan/400°F/gas mark 6.

Use a sharp knife (careful now) to slice off the top of each tomato and set aside – you'll be using these as lids, so don't make the cut too close to the top.

Using a spoon, carefully scoop out the seeds (including the juice) of each tomato and push the insides through a sieve, reserving the juice. Chop the tomato flesh.

Chop the mint leaves – the easiest way to do this is to roll the leaves up like a cigar and thinly slice.

Put the rice, feta, spring onions, mint, garlic and tomato flesh into a bowl, cover and leave to stand for 1 hour.

Stuff the tomatoes with the cold rice mixture and transfer them to a muffin tray sprayed lightly with oil – this keeps them standing up. Top with the tomato lids and bake in the oven for 30 minutes or so.

Serve with a salad.

Notes from Paul
· *This recipe is great for using up leftover risotto, if such a thing exists.*
· *Lots of supermarkets sell balsamic glazes – a little dribbled over the top of the tomatoes is very tasty indeed.*
· *If you're a bit of a klutz with a knife, pop your tomatoes into the muffin tin right from the get-go. It'll help hold the shape together.*
· *If you can't be bothered cooking the rice, just buy a pouch of instant rice from the supermarket – or swap it out for couscous.*

● ● ● ● ● ●

FETA POTATO CAKES

Serves 4
149 calories

Feta doesn't get nearly half the love it deserves, which is a shame because it's delicious. Don't worry, we know you're picking up the feta, looking at it, putting it back and getting the 'Greek Salad Cheese' instead. And why not? We do exactly the same. Look after them pennies, pet. Especially if you've just shelled out twenty quid for this book.

We're both massive fans of this one – not least because a hint of a tang from the feta and we can make believe we're sitting on a balcony somewhere hot, Shirley Valentine style, shouting nonsense at the fridge. Saying that, knowing our luck, we'd just stumble upon the island that's in Mamma Mia and we'd spend those two weeks of annual leave desperately trying to claw out our cochleas so we don't have to listen to them sing ever again. We waited for that movie to come out for months thinking it would be an absolute treat, only to have spent the subsequent however many years attempting to erase it from our memories like one might wish away a painful bout of gout. Fortunately, our lord and saviour Cher came and put everything right in 2018. And for that we must thank her.

These potato cakes are actually very tasty indeed served cold with a simple watercress salad and some decent tzatziki. Cooked chopped bacon mixed in will satisfy any meaty urges too.

600g (1lb 5oz) potatoes, peeled and chopped
1 egg
2 tablespoons fresh chives, chopped
80g (3oz/½ cup) reduced-fat feta cheese, crumbled
½ teaspoon freshly ground black pepper

Bring a large pan of salted water to the boil and add the potatoes. Boil for 15–20 minutes until tender, then drain.

Put the potatoes back into the pan and crack in an egg. Mash quickly until the egg is well combined. Add the chives, feta and pepper to the pan and continue to mash until well mixed.

Leave to cool for 15–20 minutes, then divide into 8 balls and flatten them into burger shapes.

Heat a large frying pan over a medium-high heat and spray it with a little oil. Add the potato cakes and cook for 8 minutes on each side, then serve.

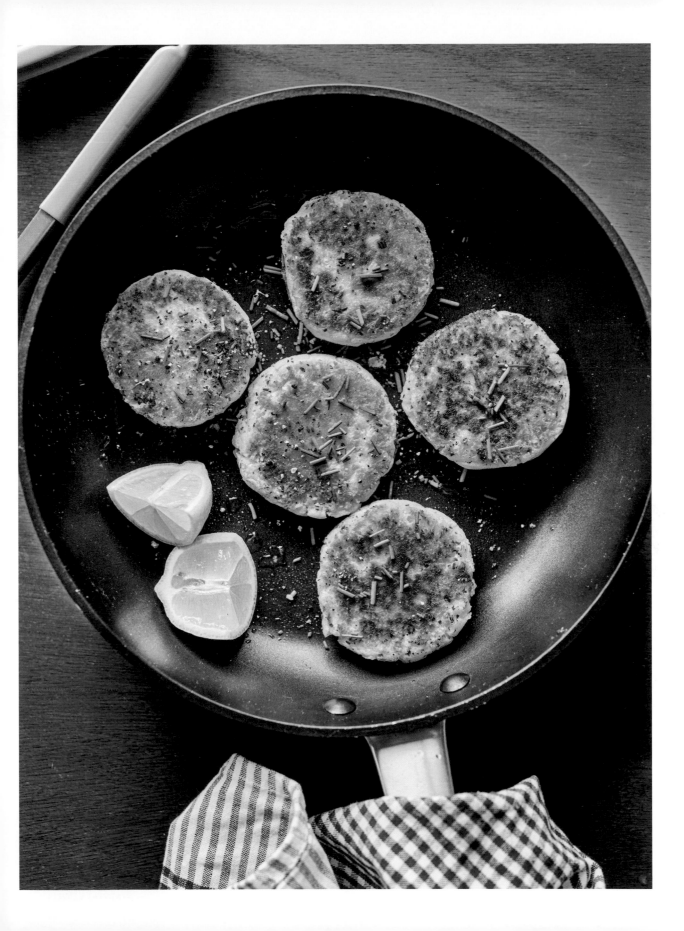

LIGHTER SPANAKOPITA? I BARELY KNEW 'ER!

Serves 4
458 calories

Spanakopita – with its layers of cheesy spinachy goodness and buttery, delicious pastry – is my absolute favourite Greek dish. Plus, let me tell you, a Geordie saying the word 'spanakopita' sounds utterly amazing, like a fridge full of syllables falling down a flight of stairs.

It's really quite a surprise that we haven't taken a holiday to Greece, given our love of the food, culture and dark baleful eyes. I'm not suggesting Paul has cause to fret taking me to the land of absolute Adonises, but I'd be shacked up with a hairy-backed farmhand before the light had faded from the fasten-your-seatbelt sign on the aeroplane. The only time Paul's thrown a plate in high emotion is when I accidentally forgot to serve his side salad directly into our kitchen bin.

It is an absolute knacker to try to make a slimming version of a spanakopita – so, although we've reduced the fat and calories in this recipe, we're using our 'a little of what you fancy does you good' motto, and combining it with the ethos that you'll probably eat two portions the same as us and at least this way it's not too deleterious to your slimming.

500g (1lb 2oz) frozen chopped spinach
1 onion, diced
2 cloves of garlic, crushed
150g (5½oz/¾ cup) cottage cheese, drained, so the curds remain
50g (1¾oz/⅓ cup) reduced-fat feta cheese
50g (1¾oz/½ cup) grated Parmesan cheese
3 eggs
a tiny pinch of nutmeg
½ teaspoon salt
½ teaspoon pepper
1 × 240g (8½oz) sheet of light puff pastry

Preheat the oven to 190°C fan/425°F/gas mark 7.

Place the spinach in a colander and run boiling water over it until fully defrosted. Once it is cool enough to touch, squeeze out as much moisture from the spinach as you can, and set aside.

Heat a small frying pan over a medium heat and spray with a little oil. Add the onion and garlic and cook for about 5 minutes, until softened.

In a bowl mix together the spinach, cottage cheese curds, feta, Parmesan, 2 eggs, nutmeg, salt and pepper.

Line a 22cm (8½ inch) baking dish with baking paper. Divide the pastry into two halves. Take one half and roll it out so that it is big enough to line the baking dish. Lay it over the dish and trim the edges. Spread over the spinach mixture. Roll out the rest of the pastry to place it on top, then crimp the edges with the back of a fork to seal. Beat the remaining egg and brush over the top to glaze.

Bake in the oven for 40 minutes, or until the pastry is bronzed and handsome, like your authors.

Notes from Paul

- *We like to serve this with a tomato and chickpea salad – take a good mixture of tomatoes, chopped with 1 large shallot, a pinch of sumac, some crushed garlic, a tablespoon each of olive oil and balsamic vinegar and some salt and pepper – leave to sit for an hour and serve warm.*
- *You can swap the puff pastry for more traditional filo. And chuck some sultanas in with the spinach and cheese too if you're feeling decadent.*

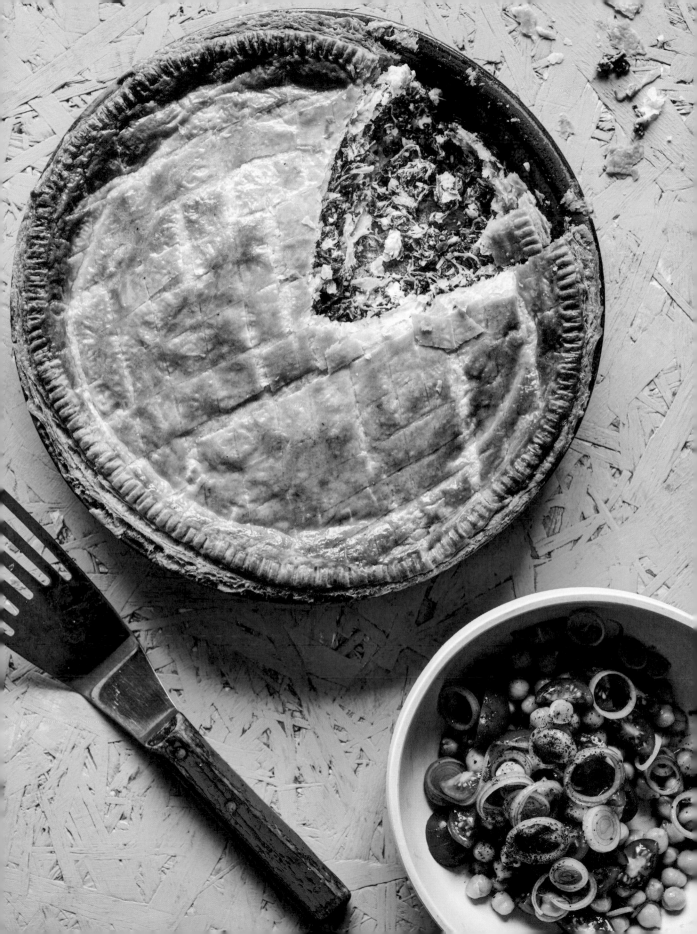

CURRY LOAF RELOADED

Serves 4
329 calories

Our very first recipe for Twochubbycubs, would you believe – though looking back it's an embarrassment of forgotten ingredients, ham-fisted instructions and a presentation that shows all the care you would expect from two men who can't afford to waste a second before eating their dinner. This has been floating around slimming classes since time immemorial and is often proffered up at 'taster nights', sliced indiscriminately by 'Sandra' (always a Sandra) who is as keen as mustard that you spend the next two hours discreetly picking eggshell out of your gums. Having been witness to as many slightly burned, wobbling, tasteless loafs as any decent human could take, we decided to make our own.

It's certainly a dish that doesn't sound terribly enchanting – we think of it almost as a vegetarian meatloaf – but it remains a go-to in our house for something quick to help ourselves to from the fridge. As with so many of our recipes, you can chuck in any stray vegetables or meat you happen to have cluttering the bottom of your fridge, their best-before-dates causing you unnecessary torment. Reduce both your waist AND your waste. Yes, that's the top calibre of writing you have come to expect, is it not?

For a final twist – hope you're sitting down now – you don't even need to make this as a loaf. Pour the uncooked mix into oiled muffin trays and you have yourself some handy grab'n'go muffins for lunch.

100g (3½oz) Indian-style packet rice
2 large leeks, sliced
1 teaspoon curry powder
1 large green pepper
1 × 400g (14oz) tin of chickpea dhal
3 eggs
5 tomatoes, diced
2 red chillies, sliced

Cook the packet rice according to the instructions and set aside.

Heat a little oil in a pan and tip in the leeks with the curry powder and sliced green pepper – you want to very gently sweat the leeks and green pepper until they soften.

Preheat the oven to 180°C fan/400°F/gas mark 6.

Mix together the chickpea dhal, eggs, tomatoes, rice, leeks and green pepper and slop the mixture into a loaf tin. Spread the sliced chillies on top of the loaf and cook in the oven for 90 minutes.

If after 90 minutes everything has set, leave to cool, then turn out on to a plate and slice into thick wedges to serve with a salad. If it needs a little longer, cover the top with tin foil and cook until firm.

This is great for a 'make on a Sunday and have during the week' dinner – it will keep in the fridge for a few days. Like a good chilli, the taste will only improve.

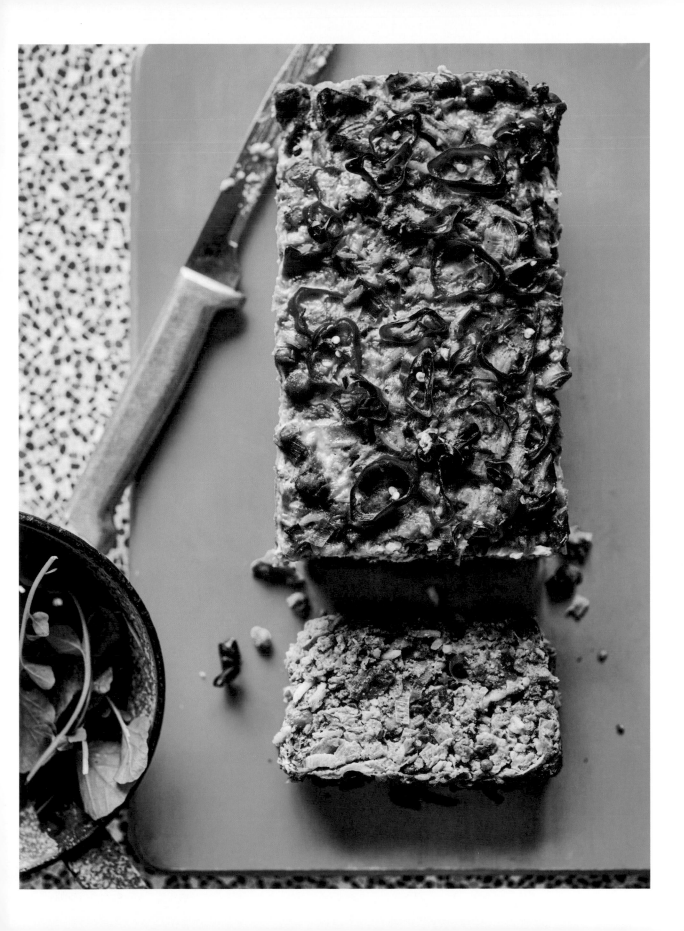

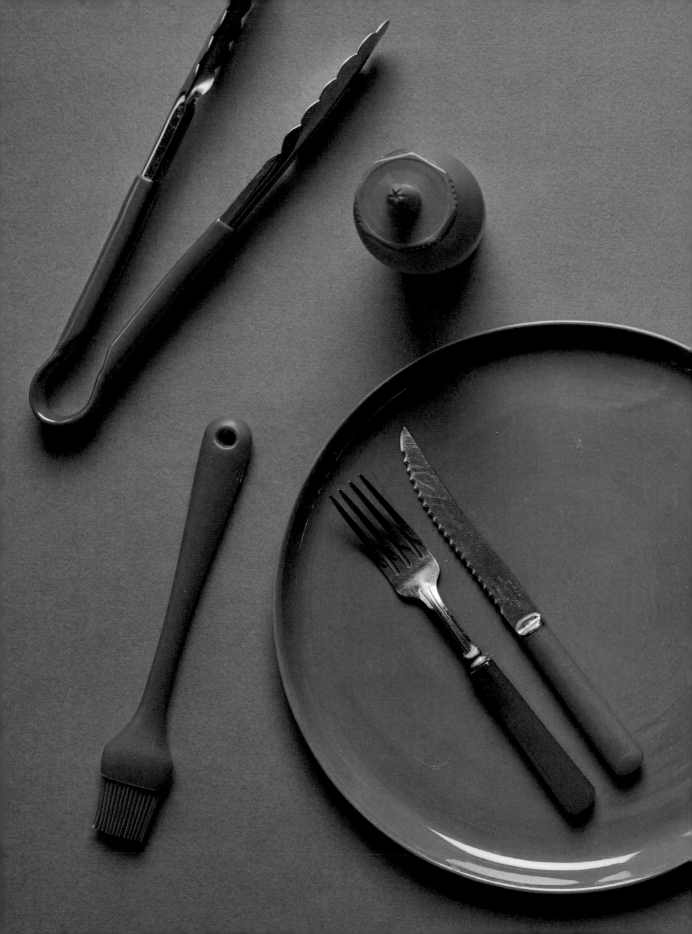

WEEKDAY DINNERS

PRAWN STIR-FRY

Serves 4
493 calories

This is an odd one for us to include because we have a hate/hate relationship with prawns here at Chubby Towers. I spent a childhood where the only prawns I'd ever see were those tiny grey/blue commas served in lurid pink sauce. Paul's exposure was limited to the four packets of Skips he had stuffed in his lunchbox, the greedy little urchin that he was.

However, here's the twist: we were given a subscription to one of those fancy recipe services where they send you a box of ingredients with a recipe card, and included – despite our stern instructions not to send us anything fishy – was a prawn stir-fry. And readers: it was delicious. Perhaps it was the way it was cooked, perhaps it was the threat of starvation facing us as we looked down at the tiny 'recommended portion size' – who can say? But there we were, aghast at ourselves for overcoming our prawn hatred, and vowed there and then to try to include prawns in our regular rotation.

Naturally, Paul threw the recipe card in the fire the very next day and so the below is an approximation built on about two years of Paul having a stab at recreating that one golden night only to be met with my grimacing face ringing our chippy in protest.

350g (12½oz) dried egg noodles
1 head of broccoli, cut into florets
2 tablespoons light soy sauce
2 tablespoons hoisin
1 tablespoon rice vinegar
1 tablespoon honey
300g (10½oz) prawns, cooked and peeled
10 cloves of garlic, crushed
5cm (2 inches) ginger, grated
2 red chillies, sliced
1 large onion, sliced
2 carrots, sliced into matchsticks
2 spring onions, sliced, to serve

Bring a large pan of water to the boil and cook the noodles according to the packet instructions. Drain the noodles and rinse under cold water, then drain again and set aside.

Meanwhile, bring another pan of water to the boil and add the broccoli. Reduce to a simmer for 4–5 minutes, until the broccoli is tender but with a bit of bite. Drain and set aside.

In a bowl, mix together the soy sauce, hoisin, rice vinegar and honey and set aside.

Heat a large frying pan over a high heat and spray with a little oil. Add the prawns to the pan and cook for 4–5 minutes, stirring frequently. Scoop them out of the pan and place in a bowl and set aside.

Spray the frying pan with some more oil, then reduce the heat to low and add the garlic, ginger and chillies. Fry for around a minute, then increase the heat to medium-high and add the onion. Fry for a few minutes, then add the carrots and fry for a further 2 minutes.

Reduce the heat to low and add a couple of tablespoons of water to the pan. Cover with a lid and cook for a few minutes. Increase the heat again to medium, and add the noodles. Stir-fry for 3–4 minutes to warm through – if they get a bit claggy, add a splash of water.

Add the sauce mixture to the pan along with the broccoli and prawns. Fry for a further 1–2 minutes, then serve, sprinkling the sliced spring onions over the top.

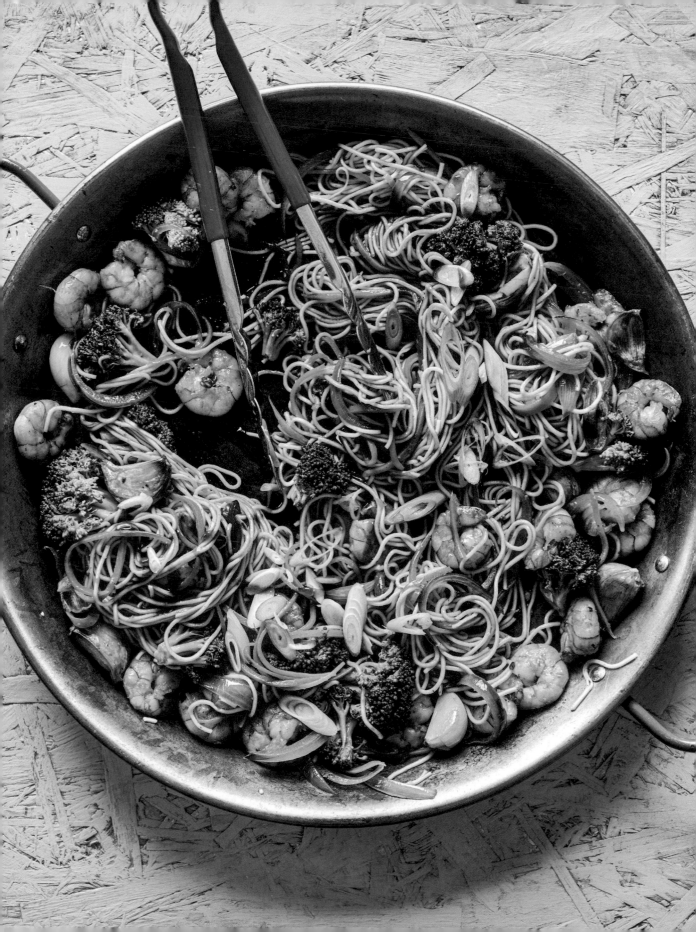

• • • • • •

THOU SHALT 'AVE A FISHY TOAST

Serves 1
462 calories

This came about when we joined an especially strict boot camp and were told, by someone whose face had never known what it was to smile, that we had to up our fish intake. I sulkily pointed out that I always had prawn crackers with my Chinese order and was met with such a furious look that I dashed home to desperately find something I could do with fish to make it faintly palatable.

I never succeeded. I don't do fish. Paul, on the other hand, will eat almost anything from the sea, and will cheerfully chomp away on anything that happens to float by. It's why we're banned from the Sealife centre – you've never lived until you've spent an hour remonstrating with a security guard while your other half picks starfish suckers off his mouth. No, I'm kidding, before you send me seafood-related hate mail – though it wouldn't be the first time I've been given something unpleasant by a postman. Blimey.

I can't in all good conscience tell you where Paul came up with this recipe – I've never asked him, because whenever he approaches me afterwards with fishy breath, it's all I can do not to fake his signature on the divorce papers and burn the house down. He does, however, assure me that it is delicious. To be fair to him, he does have excellent taste: look at the Adonis he wakes up to every morning.

This makes enough for one person, thankfully. Feel free to gussy it up, but sometimes the simplicity speaks for itself.

2 slices of good, wholemeal bread – we actually use sourdough, for the crunch
1 × 120g (4oz) tin of sardines in oil
40g (1½oz/¼ cup) light cream cheese
1 teaspoon capers, chopped
a handful of watercress
1 tablespoon lemon juice
a pinch of salt
a pinch of chilli flakes

Toast your bread – not to full 'crispiness', but just to get a bit of firmness to it.

Drain your sardines, discarding most of the oil but saving just a little to brush over your bread. Mash them with the cream cheese, chopped capers, watercress, lemon juice, salt and chilli flakes.

With your hand, make a small indentation in each slice of bread, just enough to hold your sardine mixture, and spoon it in.

Pop under the grill for a minute or 2, until piping hot and ready for action.

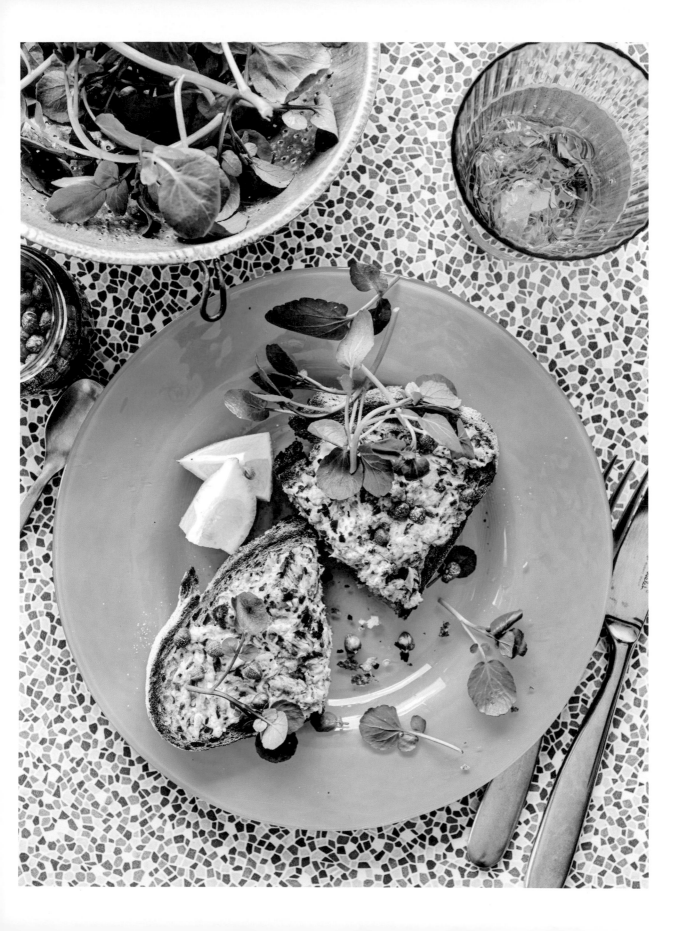

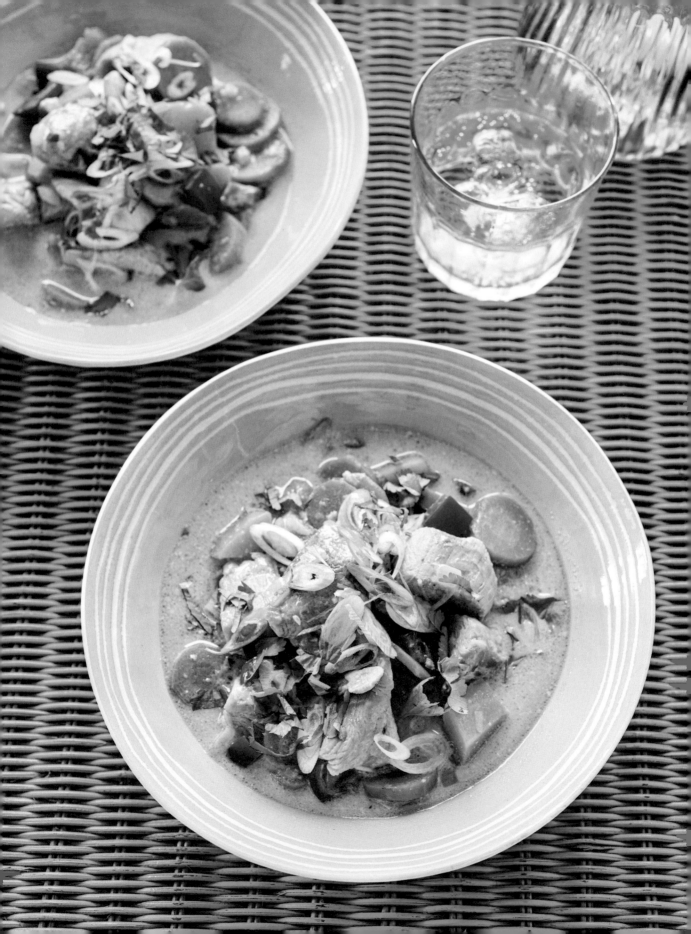

CREAMY TURKEY AUTUMN CURRY

Serves 4
343 calories

Creamy turkey autumn curry: we're only calling it 'Autumn Curry' because of the colours, we're not asking you to stir some leaves in. That would be silly indeed: we're not ones for the whole fancy presentation gimmick, as you can doubtless see from our blog. We started off with good intentions – entire cupboards in our living room are devoted to the various props and fancy serving dishes that we've bought with the intention to class up our photos. But they remain unused because as soon as the food is ready, so are we. Life's too short to be arranging cress just so on a chopping board. Don't get me wrong, we have nothing but praise for the tireless and wonderful food stylists who worked on this book; they've managed to make every dish look incredible – as opposed to our photos, which look as though the cat's already had a crack at the meal. For that we thank them endlessly.

This Autumn Curry lends itself to any vegetables you may want to chuck in – curry always does. A moment of caution: add the coconut milk slowly, lest it splits. If it does, a good stir should bring it back together but even if not, you mustn't worry, split is just tickety-boo too.

600g (1lb 5oz) turkey breast, diced
1 onion, diced
3 cloves of garlic, crushed
1 red chilli, finely diced
2.5cm (1 inch) ginger, grated
1 teaspoon ground turmeric
2 red peppers, finely diced
2 carrots, peeled and thinly sliced
1 butternut squash, peeled and chopped into 2.5cm (1 inch) cubes
250ml (9fl oz/1 cup) chicken stock
1 × 400g (14oz) tin of light coconut milk
4 spring onions, sliced, to serve
a handful of fresh coriander leaves, chopped, to serve

Heat a large frying pan over a medium heat and spray with a little oil. Add the turkey to the pan and cook until no pink remains.

Add the onion, garlic, chilli, ginger and turmeric to the pan and fry quickly for about 2 minutes, then add the peppers, carrots and butternut squash and stir.

Add the chicken stock and coconut milk, bring to the boil, and cook for about 15 minutes.

Serve in bowls, topped with the sliced spring onions and the coriander.

● ● ● ● ● ●

CHICKEN & CHORIZO RISNOTTO

Serves 4
482 calories

Risotto is one of those recipes which demands you spend your time looking moonily at the pan and stirring continuously. While this yields wonderful results, we aren't ones for standing for any longer than is absolutely necessary. Nothing says 'you're getting old' like beads of sweat on your cankles, after all. So, to minimize any sort of effort, we throw the lid on the pan, dash into the living room and pray for a good meal. This never lets us down. We call our risottos 'risnottos' because we think we're terribly clever.

The addition of chorizo may make your skin bristle, but trust us: the oil from the chorizo gives everything a lovely smoky taste without adding too many calories into the mix. You can leave it out – substitute it with peas, by all means – but why deny yourself a simple pleasure in life?

We tend to serve this on a bed of pea shoots, but that's because we're rah-rah types who listen to The Archers during dinner. Anything to drown out each other's lip-smacking noises.

4 large shallots, sliced
100g (3½oz) chorizo, diced
1 clove of garlic, crushed
2 chicken breasts, skinless and boneless, cut into 1cm (½ inch) cubes
a handful of cherry tomatoes, halved
a couple of handfuls of frozen peas
a couple of pre-cooked jarred red peppers, thinly sliced
200g (7oz/1 cup) Arborio rice
1 litre (1¾ pints/4 cups) chicken stock
100g (3½oz/½ cup) low-fat cream cheese
black pepper
20g (¾oz) grated Parmesan (optional)

Gently cook the shallots with the chorizo over a medium heat (no need to add oil – the chorizo will add its own). Add the garlic just as the onions have softened and cook for another minute.

Add the chicken and gently fry until it is almost cooked through.

Stir in the tomatoes, peas and peppers.

Add the rice and stir only enough to get some of the residual liquid over the rice. Add the stock, stir once, then clamp the lid on the pan, reduce the heat to low-medium and go entertain yourself for 20 minutes.

After 20 minutes, check – most of the liquid should have been absorbed and the rice should be lovely and soft, but if not, let it burble away for another 5 minutes or so with the lid off.

Once it's done, stir in the cream cheese and serve with plenty of black pepper and grated Parmesan, if you're fancy.

Note from Paul
If you cook this a little longer than we suggest above and really get it good and claggy, you can let it cool in the fridge and then shape it into balls for deep-frying (not one for the diet, though).

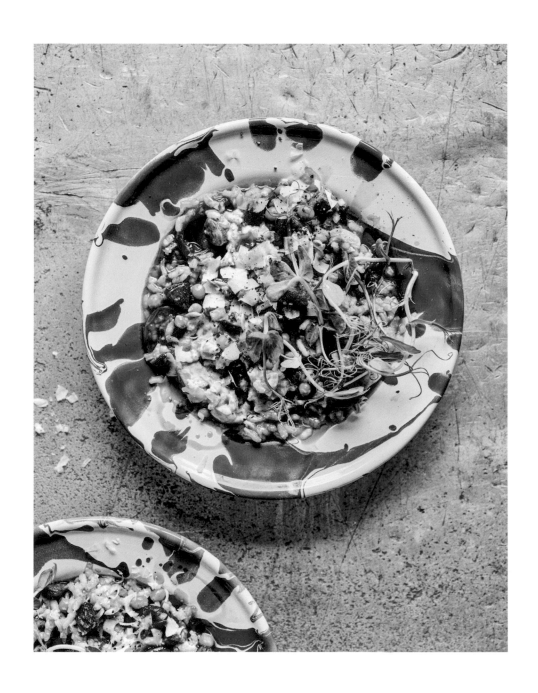

PAUL ENJOYS THIS DISH WITH A SPOONFUL
OF WHOLEGRAIN MUSTARD MIXED IN —
BUT THEN, HE ALSO ENJOYS LISTENING TO
TRACY CHAPMAN IN THE BATH, SO DON'T
TRUST A WORD HE SAYS.

FIVE MARINADES TO MAKE YOUR CHICKEN SING

• • • • •

Chicken is one of those go-to dinners, isn't it, especially when dieting. We always have a drawer full of breasts in the freezer, and not in any creepy cannibal way, you understand. If we're feeling especially virtuous, we'll pressure-cook four breasts at the start of the week, shred them with a fork, then keep the chicken in the fridge to bung into a stir-fry or a chopped salad.

More honestly, it's something for me to pick at every time I open the fridge to get the milk. I don't think I've ever managed to make a cup of tea without treating my fridge like a funeral buffet, and I'm not ashamed.

For robust dishes like a curry or a bake, we tend to use boneless chicken thighs – they lend themselves to longer cooking and stronger flavours. Save the breasts for quick dinners – sliced on top of a salad, chucked into a noodle dish. Drumsticks are Paul's personal favourite because it gives him a valid reason to get sauce all around his lips.

These marinades work well for whatever you choose – just be sure to cook your chicken thoroughly. Invest in a meat thermometer and you'll never look back. Marinate your meat for as long as you can, four hours at a minimum. The recipes cover you up until the cooking part.

Serves 2
(2 chicken drumsticks per serving)

309 calories

OOOH-ME-NIPSY CHICKEN DRUMSTICKS

Combine a few spoonfuls of fat-free Greek yoghurt with 2 tablespoons of hot chilli sauce and some chopped mint leaves. Put everything into a sandwich bag, making sure every last bit is covered with sauce, and leave in the fridge until you're ready, taking the opportunity to tumble them about when you pass.

Serves 2
(1 chicken breast per serving)

235 calories

TICKLE-ME-PICKLE

This one you're going to have to trust us on – and it works better with chicken breasts, but drumsticks will do just fine. Take a jar of pickled gherkins and slice up a few of the larger ones, saving the rest for a salad or to slip into burgers for people you don't like. Tip the breasts and plenty of the pickle juice into a sandwich bag and leave to marinate for a few hours.

Serves 2
(2 chicken drumsticks
per serving)

204 calories

Serves 4
(2 chicken drumsticks
per serving)

291 calories

Serves 4
(2 chicken drumsticks
per serving)

228 calories

DILF-STICKS

These Drumsticks I Love Featuring at dinner are so-called because
the recipe is full of salt and pepper – why else? Combine 2 tablespoons
of sea salt with a tablespoon of freshly ground black pepper. Spray
your chicken with olive oil, then rub that salt and pepper into every
nook and cranny – you're not aiming for total coverage, don't fret –
and shake off any excess. Grill when you're ready, turning the chicken
halfway through.

OH HONEY CHICKEN

Mix together 4 tablespoons of honey with a tablespoon of decent
wholegrain mustard and 2 tablespoons of olive oil and, again, pop
everything into a sandwich bag and tumble it around. You might fret
about the amount of honey and oil if you're watching your waistline,
but don't – a little goes a very long way in this recipe.

HERBY TART

Combine 2 tablespoons of lemon zest with 120ml (4fl oz/½ cup)
of lemon juice (fresh, mind you) and 2 tablespoons of olive oil.
Add 2 tablespoons of fresh oregano (or dried, if you're lazy) and
a few good pinches of salt and pepper.

●●○○●●

STUFFED YORKSHIRE PUDDING WRAPS

Makes 2 large wraps

495 calories with chicken, stuffing and gravy

1 tablespoon olive oil
30g (1oz/3 tablespoons)
    plain flour
2 eggs
75ml (2½fl oz/⅓ cup)
    semi-skimmed milk
a tiny pinch of salt
a pinch of garlic powder

We're not one for food fads and fussy eating; however, we were all too eager to jump on the Yorkshire pudding wrap bus. I shared a Yorkshire pudding wrap with a good friend of mine back one lusty summer day and it was just like that scene in Lady and the Tramp *where the dogs share the spaghetti, only our scene ends with him threatening to glass me if I took the last roast potato. How I laughed through my bruising.*

This recipe gives you the basics and an idea for fillings, but honestly, use anything you like. We've seen a sweet take on this with ice-cream, Nutella and someone to bring you round from your sugar coma moments later, but we'll stick to savoury, thank you very much.

Note: these won't rise like your average Yorkie, but will rather stay fairly flat. Which is good for rolling.

Preheat the oven to 220°C fan/475°F/gas mark 9.

You'll need a couple of small, standard circular cake tins. Use a brush to oil the tins, or simply spray them with a good olive oil spray. Pop them into the oven to get nice and hot.

Blend together the flour, eggs, milk, salt and garlic powder – we use a stand-up blender for this but you can do it by hand – whisk furiously, mind, no lumps.

Once the pans are hot, pour half the mix into one tin and half into the other and pop them into the oven. They take about 5 minutes, maybe a bit longer – just keep an eye on them and once they're browned and set, take them out of the oven.

Let them cool but not for too long – if you 'roll' them while they're warm and keep them like that while they cool, it'll make your life easier down the line.

Once it's time to plate up, unroll the wraps, fill with whatever you like, then roll up and serve with gravy.

FILLING IDEAS

The obvious answer is to use whatever leftovers you have from the Sunday roast, or, as we call it here at Chubby Towers, the evening meal. Shredded chicken, stuffing and gravy is a winner.

Go veggie by roasting a load of parsnips and carrots – keeping some crunch to them – in honey.

Roast beef spread with a little horseradish sauce and, again, doused with gravy is delicious.

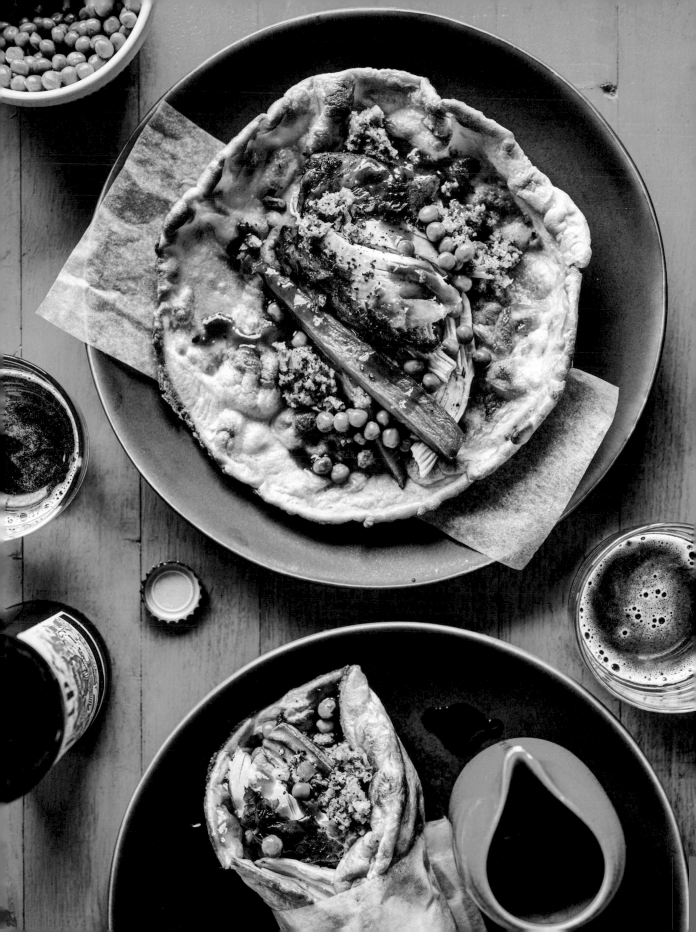

HAM & PINEAPPLE PASTA BAKE

Serves 6
475 calories

We originally called this a 'Hawaiian bake' until we realized that 'Hawaiian' is how my very Geordie mother used to call her children back from working up the chimneys. We're joking – she used to send us down the mines. We appreciate that the addition of pineapple in a pasta bake sounds like madness, but trust us: the sweetness of the fruit adds another layer of loveliness into what is an already tasty dish. It freezes well too – so keep some aside in the freezer for those days when all you want to do is rush home and rest your bunions, which, if you're like us, is every single day.

Before we get to the recipe, you may be thinking about where we stand on the pineapple on a pizza issue – it's terrifically simple. Anyone who puts pineapple on a pizza should be sent to the foot of the stairs. The only thing that belongs on a pizza is my sweet lips.

350g (12½oz/3½ cups) dried pasta – any pasta will do, we're not sitting in judgement here
300g (10½oz) bacon medallions
4 thick slices of good ham, cut into chunks
230g (8oz/1½ cups) pineapple chunks – fresh is better, but we sometimes buy the pre-cut fruit from the supermarket if we're feeling especially lazy
750g (1½ lb/3 cups) passata
150g (5½oz/1½ cups) mozzarella
80g (3oz/¾ cup) grated extra mature Cheddar cheese, for the top (optional, but why deprive yourself?)

Preheat the oven to 180°C fan/400°F/gas mark 6.

Cook your pasta according to the packet instructions.

Meanwhile, grill the bacon until it's cooked – but you want it soft and tasty, not like shoe leather. Once the bacon is cooked, cut it into chunks.

Mix the cooked pasta, ham and bacon chunks, pineapple and passata together in a large pan, then tip it into an ovenproof dish.

Dot the bake with chunks of mozzarella, then, if you're using it, scatter the grated Cheddar over the top. Don't be tempted to add salt – the bacon will provide plenty of that.

Cook in the oven for about 20 minutes, then finish it off under the grill so the cheese starts bubbling.

Serve with a light salad on the side to pointedly ignore.

Notes from Paul
- This is what we consider a 'scalable' recipe – you can easily double or triple the ingredients (though you'll need a big oven) to make plenty of leftovers for lunches and evening meals.
- While we normally recommend salting the pasta water, we tend not to do so for this dish, as the bacon adds a salty flavour.

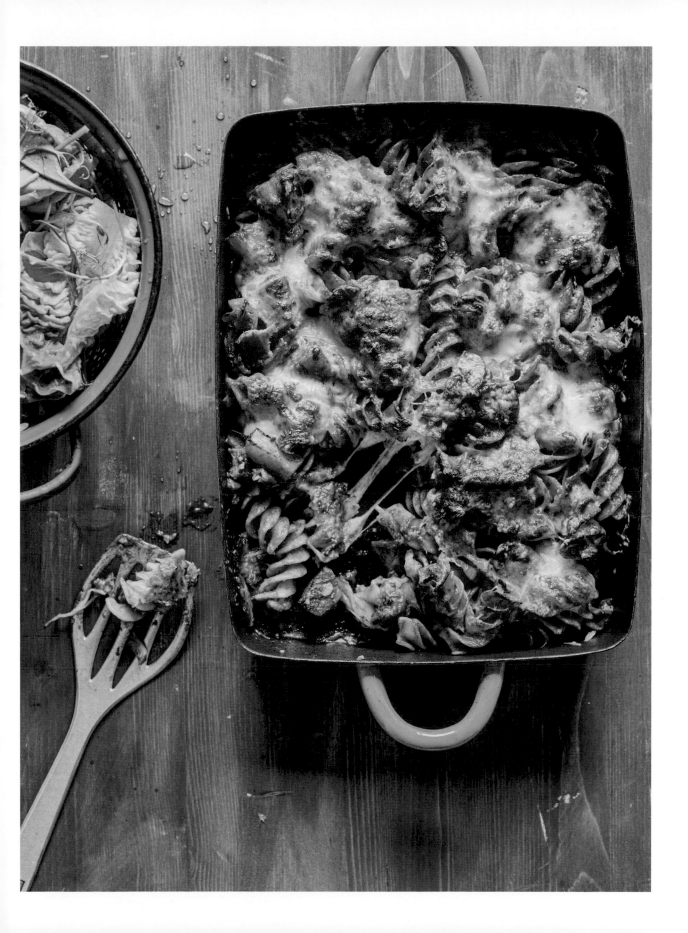

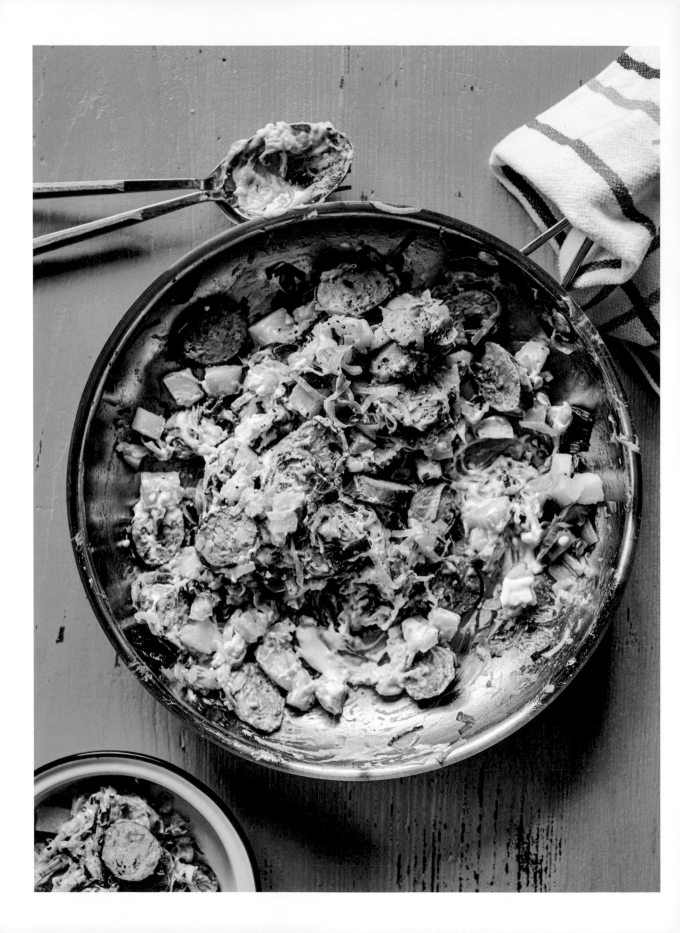

● ● ● ● ● ●

ONE-POT CREAMY LEEK & SAUSAGE BAKE

Serves 4
380 calories

6 good-quality sausages
500g (1lb 2oz) leeks, finely sliced
1 large white onion, thinly sliced
a pinch of salt
100ml (3½fl oz/½ cup) white wine
100ml (3½fl oz/½ cup) good chicken stock
a couple of large potatoes, peeled and finely diced like, well, dice
100g (3½oz/½ cup) extra-light cream cheese
freshly ground black pepper

This is another recipe that we picked up from our gallivanting – this time from Switzerland, a place so beautiful that every turn of the train track took my breath away. Mind, that was usually because Paul had returned with the coffees and presented me with a bill so significant that it made me ponder whether he'd bought shares in the rail company. If you haven't been, you simply must: one of the highlights of the trip was eating fondue for six in a chalet for two high up in the Alps.

So much Swiss cuisine seems to revolve around the addition of cheese and cream into every conceivable meal, which is tricky when you're cutting down, but we just had to bring a recipe over for this book. We tried making fondue healthy but there's absolutely no way, though I'm sure there's a Dismal Debbie out there currently forcing her children to eat molten quark with a manic grin on her face. So, apologies for that, but please enjoy our healthier take on a classic Swiss recipe with our best intentions.

You'll need a good deep non-stick frying pan for this.

We like to dry-fry the sausages first, so the fat from the sausages gets into the pan (if you're using very low-fat sausages, use a bit of oil) – so do this, then set aside the sausages until later.

With the sausages done, gently fry the leeks and onion in the fat from the sausage with a pinch of salt. After about 5 minutes, throw the heat up, chuck in the white wine (to deglaze the pan), then reduce the heat again, add the stock and cover for another 5 minutes.

Finely slice the sausages and add them to the pan together with the cubed potatoes. Let everything simmer gently for around 15 minutes, or until the potatoes have cooked – add a touch more stock if things are looking dry, although there shouldn't be a great amount of liquid.

When you're ready to serve, stir in the cream cheese, season with plenty of black pepper, and enjoy.

Notes from Paul
- *Grated Gruyère cheese stirred in towards the end lifts this dish into heavenly status.*
- *Don't be tempted to buy those pre-sliced leeks unless you absolutely have to – they'll be too thick for this dish.*
- *A mandolin slicer will make quick work of slicing both the leeks and the onion, plus your fingers too if you're not careful.*
- *If you're not a fan of white wine you can leave it out, though don't take it out just to save a few calories – it'll bubble off merrily of its own accord.*

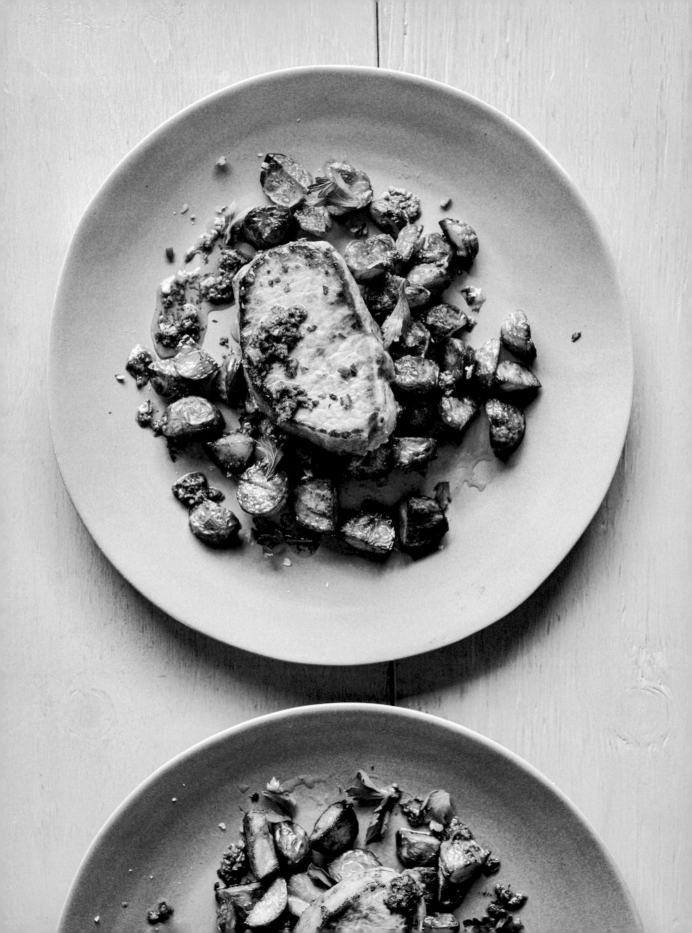

PORK MEDALLIONS WITH A CHIMICHURRI SAUCE

Serves 4
331 calories

Chimichurri is an underrated sauce – you can keep your gelatinous gloopy pepper sauces and fancy-pants béarnaise, thank you all the same – the addition of a load of fresh, zippy herbs and garlic will never be a terrible thing. You can go two routes here: buy the medallions already chopped and ready to go, or spend a little money and get yourself a pork tenderloin. This works for two reasons – you can slice your chops as thick as you like and you get to make tiresome 'well just LOOK at the length of my pork' jokes in the supermarket, until you realize your significant other hasn't only distanced himself from you, but has paid for the shopping, driven home and started looking at express divorces.

There's a terrific recipe on our blog for a strawberry and balsamic glaze that we also use for pork and we encourage you to take a look if you're in the mood for something a little fruitier.

Fresh herbs are the key here – this just won't be the same if you're using some green dust that you've had lurking in the back of the cupboard since the Queen's coronation. Why not start a little herb garden in your kitchen? Once you've set away a few plants on the windowsill and taken a bit of time to get them established, you'll never go back.

500g (1lb 2oz) new potatoes, quartered
3 tablespoons olive oil
4 pork medallions
30g (1oz/1 cup) fresh parsley leaves
30g (1oz/1 cup) fresh coriander leaves
3 cloves of garlic, crushed
1 green chilli, deseeded
2 tablespoons white wine vinegar

Preheat the oven to 220°C fan/475°F/gas mark 9.

Place the new potatoes in a small roasting tin and drizzle with 1 tablespoon of the olive oil. Tumble well to ensure that all the potatoes are coated. Roast in the oven for 25 minutes.

Heat a large frying pan over a medium-high heat and spray with a little oil. Add the pork medallions to the pan and cook for 3 minutes on each side. Transfer to a plate to rest.

Put the parsley, coriander, garlic, chilli, the remaining 2 tablespoons of olive oil and the white wine vinegar into a food processor and pulse until combined.

Serve the pork with the potatoes and drizzle over the chimichurri sauce.

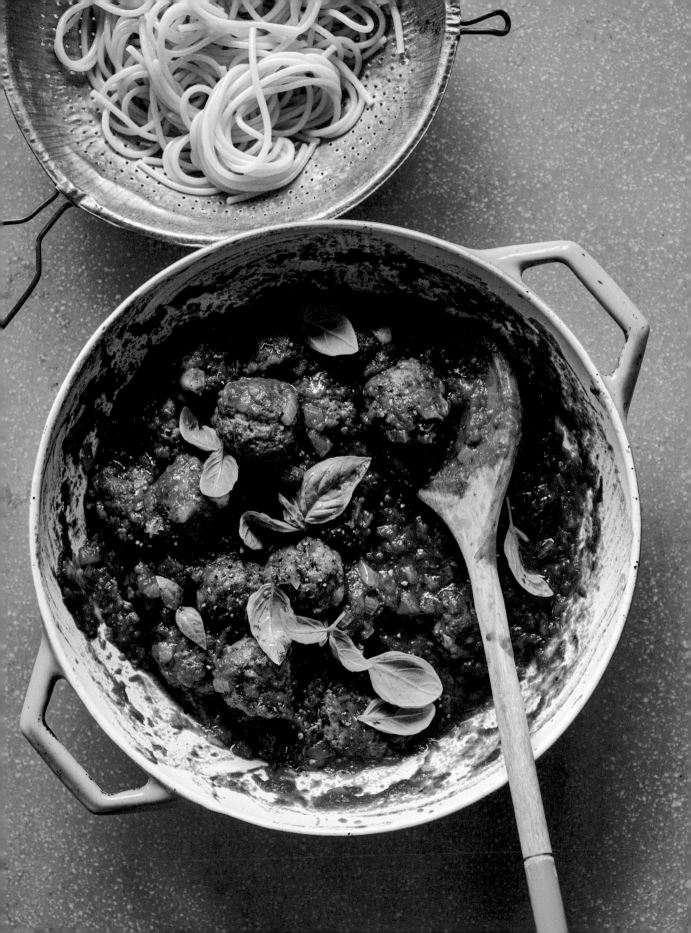

LAMB & HALLOUMI MEATBALLS

Serves 4
399 calories

Meatballs have been an absolute staple of our blog – partly because they're such an easy dish, partly because they're always good fun to make. On the blog you'll find recipes for meatballs cooked in Guinness, buffalo chicken meatballs and my own personal favourite: our hot take on IKEA meatballs.

To be honest, it's just a luxury to enjoy a whole plate of IKEA meatballs without the boiling rage of an ongoing argument spoiling the taste. Has anyone ever managed to navigate a trip around IKEA without their marriage falling apart like soggy cake? The three months when Paul and I were designing our own kitchen and ending up in IKEA at least twice a week were dark days indeed – we've weathered the storms of infidelity far more smoothly than trying to choose the correct handles for our drawers. It was lucky that Paul was able to storm off into the bedroom department and sob into a show pillow otherwise he would never have got it out of his system.

Don't be afraid of lamb mince – it does indeed have a higher fat content than the likes of pork mince or turkey mince, but the fat adds the flavour. You can lower the fat content by having a butcher make the mince up for you: never be afraid to make friends with your local butcher. Our butcher loves the sight of us – I think we've paid for his caravan twice over.

500g (1lb 2oz) lamb mince
125g (4½oz) halloumi cheese, diced into small cubes
2 teaspoons dried oregano
1 teaspoon paprika
1 onion, finely diced
3 cloves of garlic, crushed
1 × 400g (14oz) tin of chopped tomatoes
2 tablespoons tomato purée
150ml (5fl oz/⅔ cup) chicken stock
8 fresh basil leaves

Preheat the oven to 200°C fan/425°F/gas mark 7.

Mix together the lamb mince, halloumi, 1 teaspoon of oregano and the paprika, being careful not to over-mix.

Divide the mixture into 20–24 portions and roll them into meatballs.

Spray a large baking sheet with a little oil and place the meatballs on the sheet. Bake in the oven for 20 minutes.

Meanwhile, place a large saucepan over a medium heat, spray with a little oil and add the onion. Cook for 2–3 minutes, until it is starting to turn translucent. Add the garlic and stir well, then add the rest of the ingredients to the pan. Bring to the boil, then reduce the heat and simmer for 10–15 minutes, until thickened.

When the meatballs are ready, add them to the pan and cook for another 10 minutes.

● ● ● ● ● ●

PESTO LAMB STEAKS

Serves 4
320 calories

Pesto lamb: one of the quickest dinner ideas you'll ever make – and with quite a bit of perfect timing and/or judicious editing, the story relates tangentially to the recipe. Makes a change.

See, I'm writing this recipe up after quite the tumultuous day with our youngest child, Bowser. He's the most affectionate cat you can imagine when he's with us but by goodness, he makes up for it when he goes outside. He's the type of cat that would pick a fight with an articulated lorry and come back with blood on his paws and a winning smile. That's great, although I confess it can be frustrating being emasculated by your own cat. Over the last few years he has lost half of one ear, shredded the other, almost lost an eye, broken his tail and had a tooth knocked out.

The reason I mention Bowser? He has a thing for lamb. I say a thing: Paul and I spent an hour studding a massive lamb joint with lemon, rosemary and garlic slivers, anointing it with herbed oil, and then cooked it low and slow for a good few hours. Taking it out of the oven to rest, we took a fifteen minute break – came back in to find the entire joint on the floor with the cat hacking away at it. Fuming? His lips certainly were. So, if you're making this gorgeous pesto lamb, and really you ought to be at least thinking about it at this point, keep it away from your cat. Or mine.

25g (1oz/1 cup) fresh basil leaves
2 tablespoons grated Parmesan
    cheese
1 teaspoon olive oil
2 cloves of garlic
1 tablespoon lemon juice
¼ teaspoon salt
¼ teaspoon freshly ground black
    pepper
4 lamb leg steaks

Preheat the grill to medium-high.

In a food processor or mini-chopper, mix the basil leaves, Parmesan, olive oil, garlic, lemon juice, salt and pepper to make a smooth pesto.

Lay the lamb steaks out on a grill pan and spoon half the pesto over the top. Place under the grill and cook for 3–5 minutes.

Turn the steaks over and spoon over the remaining pesto. Cook for a further 3–5 minutes.

Remove from the grill and leave to rest on a warm plate for 5 minutes

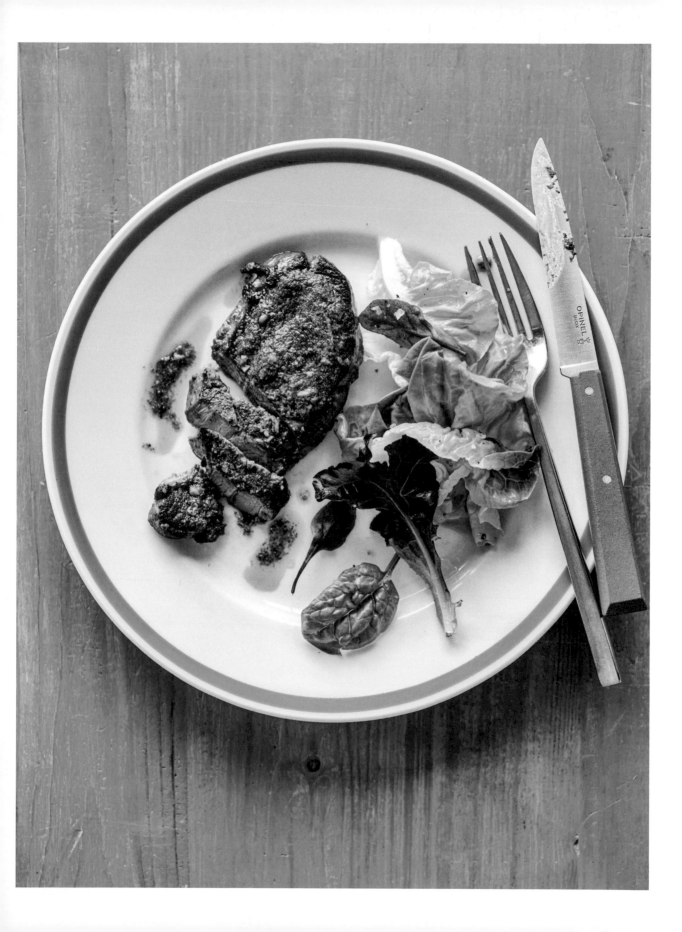

PROPER HEARTY BEEF & VEGETABLE SOUP

Serves 4
381 calories

Having covered Bowser in the previous recipe, it seems only fair to mention the other cat, Sola. Sola is the antithesis of Bowser: where he knows how to love, she only knows how to harm. I can count on one severely-shredded hand the amount of times she has let us pick her up without her deciding the best escape route is directly through my major arteries. You don't own a cat – they own you – and never has this been more evident than in this tortoiseshell bundle of 'joy'.

She doesn't even have good cause to be so permanently angry: she has a cat bed hanging from the radiator, a fresh-water fountain for her dainty ways and all manner of toys that she has batted under the sofa and promptly ignored. We stopped buying the off-brand cat food when she protested by taking a dump in the shower. We even rescued her from a cat and dog shelter! Tsk. The only time she has ever shown us love is when we took her to get her tubes tied – she came back badly shaved, bleeding and groggy from being put under (I must get that vet's personal number).

She's getting old now, and I'm fairly sure the time will come when she rolls a seven and crosses that rainbow bridge to the land of god-awful metaphors. Let me make you a guarantee – I'll bet my house on this – when she does perish, she will do so somewhere incredibly awkward, like in the door frame of our bathroom. This'll mean her final act on Earth will be tripping me up so I crack my head on the toilet. Only then will her soul rest.

400g (14oz) diced beef
1 onion, finely diced
2 cloves of garlic, crushed
1 potato, cut into 1cm cubes
4 carrots, thinly sliced
2 celery stalks, sliced
1 litre (1¾ pints/4 cups) beef stock
1 × 400g (14oz) tin of chopped tomatoes
500g (1lb 2oz/2 cups) passata
2 tablespoons tomato purée
1 teaspoon dried oregano
½ teaspoon dried basil
¼ teaspoon dried thyme
½ teaspoon salt
½ teaspoon freshly ground black pepper
¼ of a cabbage, roughly chopped

Heat a large pan over a medium-high heat and spray with a little oil. Add the beef and the onions and cook until the beef has browned.

Add the garlic to the pan and stir for 1 minute, then add everything else except for the cabbage. Increase the heat to high and bring to the boil, then reduce to a simmer and cook for 15–20 minutes.

Add the cabbage, cook for a further 5 minutes, and serve.

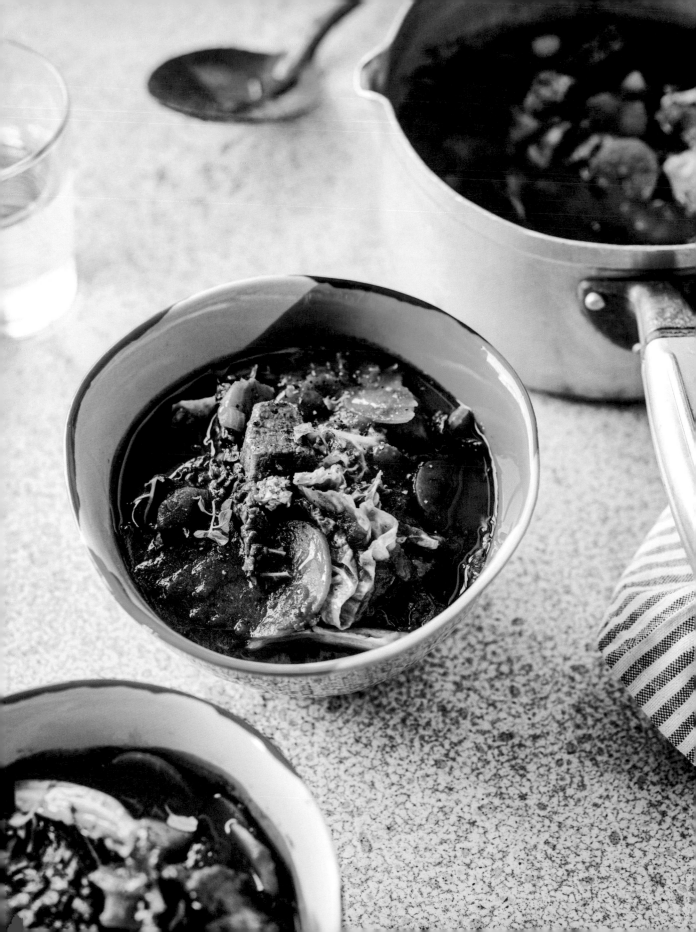

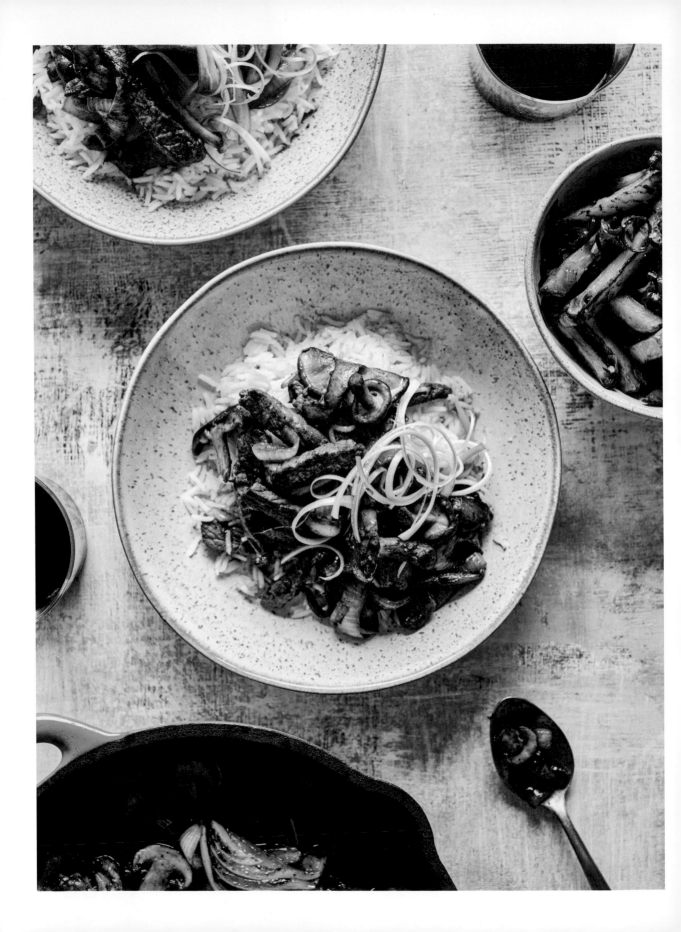

DATE-WRECKING GARLIC BEEF

Serves 4
259 calories

2 tablespoons soy sauce
2 tablespoons lime juice
1 tablespoon fish sauce
6 cloves of garlic, crushed
a pinch of salt and black pepper
500g (1lb 2oz) beef strips
1 × 200g (7oz) pack of
    mushrooms, sliced – try to
    choose an exotic mix
1 onion, thickly sliced
2 spring onions, sliced, to garnish

There's a terrific Nigella Lawson recipe that uses about thirty cloves of garlic and guarantees that people will be standing about two miles downwind of you for a good few days. That inspired this recipe, which also uses a frightening amount of garlic but tastes absolutely fine. By cooking the garlic a little, you take away that honking smell and are left with a smooth, mellow flavour that lifts this otherwise simple dish. That said, we call this our date-wrecking beef for good reason. Serve with a shot of Listerine on the side, that's all we will say.

Our first date wasn't especially memorable – I turned up at Paul's house with a bunch of flowers because he wasn't very well, and we proceeded to do exactly what you'd expect two young gay men in the first flush of lust to do. Watched Family Guy, *fell asleep. It was only when Paul broke wind so loudly in his sleep that he woke me up that I knew he was the one for me. Fun fact: on our second date, Paul came back to my house in Newcastle, and never went back to his house in Portsmouth. Who could blame him? I had name-brand crisps and a Wii; he had a packet of fish fingers and a rent deficit. There's a glorious picture of us cuddled up on our games room wall – I'm looking into the camera with eyes full of love, he's looking over my shoulder at my wallet sitting on the table.*

Ah, young love. This is the moment in the book where I say we're still hopelessly in love and the romance never died.

In a bowl, mix together the liquids. In another bowl, mix together the garlic with the salt and pepper to make a paste.

Spray a frying pan with a little oil. Over a high heat, fry the beef and mushrooms until brown, then remove them from the pan and set aside.

Add the onions to the same pan and cook for about 5–10 minutes, stirring constantly, until they start to turn golden. Add the garlic paste to the onions, making sure it doesn't stick to the pan.

Return the beef and mushrooms to the pan and stir well to combine. Add the sauce mixture and get everything coated and sticky.

Serve with rice and garnish with spring onions.

Note from Paul
Mushrooms are one of those foods that many people say they don't like, but they've grown up on button mushrooms – try an exotic mix from the supermarket instead, finely sliced – the taste is so different. If you're still not sold, swap them for more beef, or add some sliced red peppers.

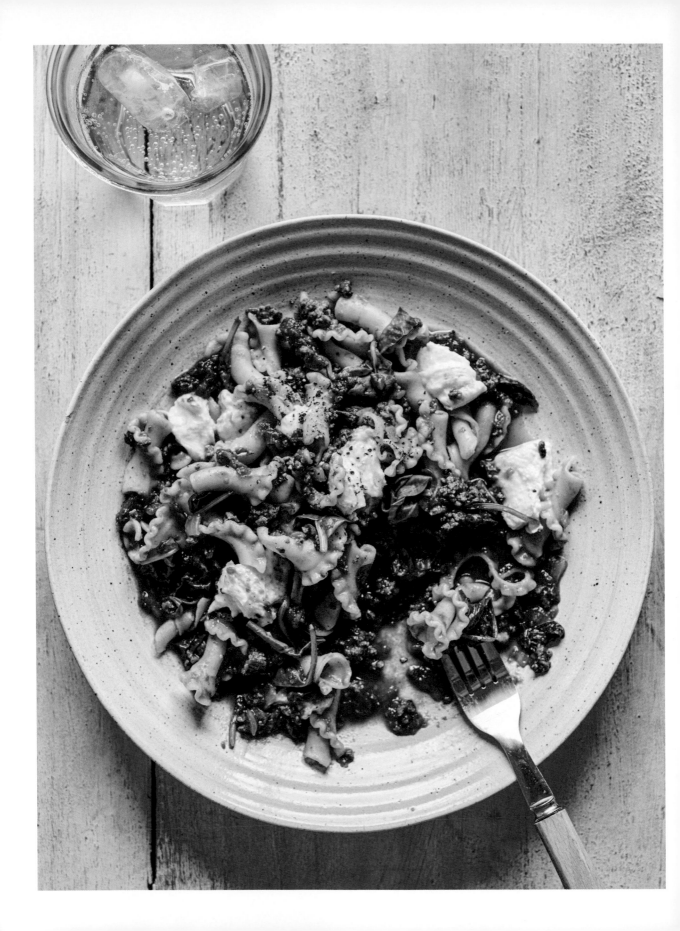

CHEAT'S LASAGNE

●　●　●　●　●　●

Serves 4
498 calories

370g (13oz) lean beef mince
3 cloves of garlic, crushed
1 large onion, finely chopped
250g (9oz/1 cup) passata
1 × 400g (14oz) tin of chopped
    tomatoes
500ml (18fl oz/2 cups) beef stock
6 big handfuls of spinach
1 tablespoon dried mixed herbs
200g (7oz/2 cups) dried pasta
    (we used gigli pasta, but only
    because we're very live, laugh,
    love in this household)
125g (4½oz/1 cup) light
    mozzarella, torn into small
    chunks
freshly ground black pepper
20g (¾oz/1¼ cup) grated
    Parmesan cheese, to serve

We call this dish 'cheat's lasagne' because I cooked it to try to make it up to Paul when he realized the milkman was coming to our house three times a day. The signs were there: the empty milk bottles on the step, the £400-a-week dairy bill, the fact that I'm lactose intolerant, but Paul is about as sharp as a bowling ball and a little slow on the uptake.

I jest, of course. This is a 'cheat's lasagne' simply because it tastes like a lasagne but without the need to set aside four days to build it. We have seen all manner of white sauce 'alternatives' (fnar fnar) during our time writing Twochubbycubs and they've all been uniformly awful. Any time you're asked to add yoghurt and quark, the best thing to do is to pop it straight in the bin.

Find yourself a nice large casserole pan and fry the mince with a few sprays of oil.

Add the garlic and onion and cook for another few minutes, then add the passata, tinned tomatoes, stock, spinach, herbs and pasta and give everything a stir. Bring to the boil, then reduce to a simmer and cover with a lid. Cook for about 15 minutes, until the pasta is al dente.

Add the mozzarella to the pan and stir through until melted.

Serve in a nice big bowl, sprinkled with the grated Parmesan and plenty of black pepper.

Notes from Paul
· *Add some chilli flakes to the pan when you're cooking the onions if you like a bit of fire in your belly.*
· *If you fancy making this more into a 'lasagne', pop the cooked pasta and the sauce into a Pyrex dish and top with a white sauce.*

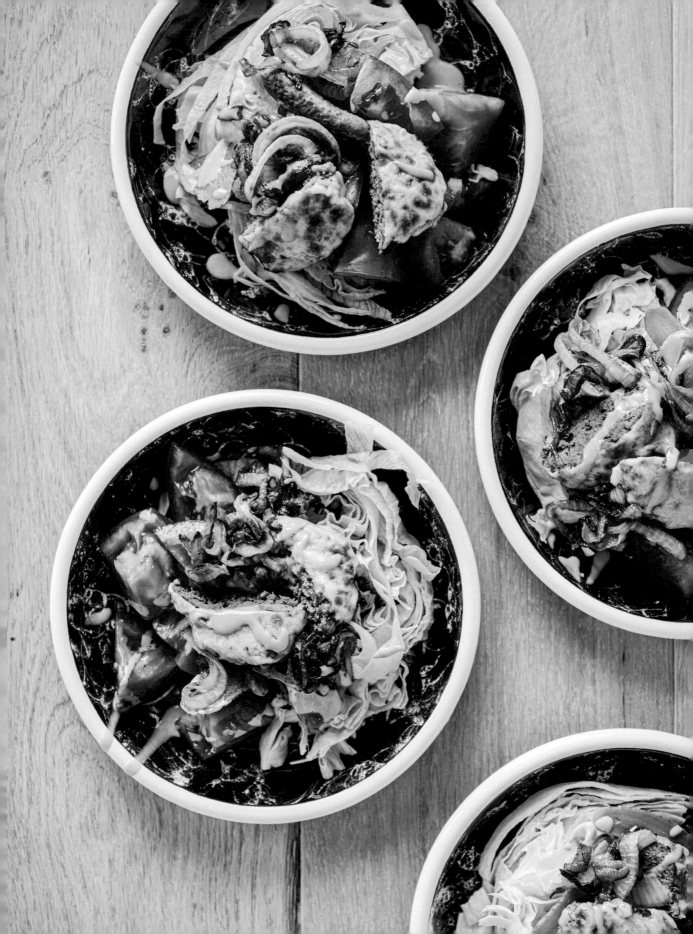

CHEESEBURGER SALAD

Serves 4
403 calories

I'm a big fan of the title of this recipe: cheeseburger salad. I mean, can you think of two words that don't belong next to each other more than those? Happy marriage doesn't count, that's a given. We've taken all the worst bits of a salad (i.e. having a salad) and combined it with something delicious and wonderful (i.e. having a cheeseburger).

We picked up the idea for this dish in Paris a couple of years ago, and it appears regularly on our rotation whenever we can't be fussed making something fancy or Paul has forsaken bread because that's what makes him fat, not the après-work McDonald's, you understand.

We had spent the morning wandering around the catacombs under Paris, leaving us starving and exhausted. Which to be fair is our status-quo anyway, but please, factor in blisters. We skedaddled into the first restaurant we found without taking pause to check the menu and ordered the first two dishes my finger fell upon. So cultured. Paul had a pizza, I had a salad – this cheeseburger salad, no less. Get it made.

500g (1lb 2oz) lean beef mince
4 × 40g (1½oz) slices of reduced-fat Cheddar cheese
1 large onion, sliced
1 iceberg lettuce, chopped
4 large tomatoes, cut into chunks
20 gherkins, sliced
4 tablespoons reduced-fat Thousand Island dressing

Divide the beef mince into 4 portions. Roll each one into a ball, then squash down into a rough burger shape.

Heat a large frying pan over a medium-high heat and spray with a little oil. Fry the burgers for 3–4 minutes, then flip them over and top each one with a slice of cheese. Fry for a further 3–4 minutes, then remove to a plate to rest. Add the onion to the pan and fry for 7–8 minutes.

Fill 4 bowls or plates with the chopped lettuce, topped with tomato chunks, gherkins and fried onions.

Roughly chop the burgers and add them to the bowls. Drizzle over a tablespoon per bowl of the Thousand Island dressing, and eat.

Notes from Paul

· *For a bit of crunch you can crush up half a bag of tortillas and sprinkle them over the top.*
· *You can make your own Thousand Island dressing by mixing together 1 tablespoon of crème fraîche, 1 tablespoon of reduced-fat mayonnaise, 1 tablespoon of natural yoghurt, ½ teaspoon of paprika, 2 teaspoons of mustard, 2 teaspoons of tomato purée and 1 teaspoon of white wine vinegar.*

FIVE-ALARM CHILLI

• • • • • •

Serves 4
384 calories

250g (9oz) lean beef mince
250g (9oz) pork mince
5 cloves of garlic, crushed
1 large onion, diced
125ml (4fl oz/½ cup) stout
1 red pepper, diced
5 mixed chillies, diced
    (with seeds!)
1 × 400g (14oz) tin of kidney
    beans, drained and rinsed
1 × 400g (14oz) tin of tomatoes
1 × 198g (7oz) tin of sweetcorn
1 tablespoon hot chilli powder
1 tablespoon paprika
2 teaspoons garlic powder
2 teaspoons ground black pepper
1 tablespoon ground cumin
1 × 15g (½ oz) sachet of hot
    seasoning mix (see notes)
1 tablespoon curry powder
125ml (4fl oz/½ cup) black coffee
2 tablespoons cider vinegar
1 tablespoon tomato sauce
1 tablespoon barbecue sauce
1 tablespoon Worcestershire
    sauce
1 tablespoon sriracha
2 teaspoons soy sauce

To serve
4 tablespoons crème fraîche
2 spring onions, sliced
a handful of fresh coriander
    leaves, chopped

Confession time: we stole the title for this from The Simpsons, *namely the episode where Homer goes to a chilli cook-off and ends up eating such a strong pepper that he hallucinates all manner of trippy scenes and realizes Marge is his soulmate. Look, I'm an absolute sucker for a love story involving food – it's pretty much my raison d'être.*

Chilli is one of those foods that divide Chubby Towers, however, and can lead to all sorts of sulking and titty lipping. See, Paul likes his food mild and inoffensive – just like him – whereas I like to spend the next day crying into a chilled toilet roll. That aside, this chilli seems to satisfy us both.

Put a large heavy-bottomed casserole pan over a medium heat and spray it with oil. Add the mince and let it brown, then add the garlic and onion and cook until no pink meat remains.

Add the stout to the pan and stir to deglaze, then add the rest of the ingredients. Cook on medium-high for 5–10 minutes, then reduce to barely a simmer and continue to cook on the lowest possible heat for 4–5 hours, stirring occasionally and checking to make sure it hasn't dried out.

Stir, and serve topped with the crème fraîche, spring onions and coriander leaves.

Notes from Paul
- *You don't have to use both pork and beef, but using both does add to the flavour. You can use whichever one you have.*
- *Make this the day before if you can. The longer a chilli can sit and soak up its own flavours, the better.*
- *Don't be afraid to use whatever you have in this – we chucked in a lot of what we had lying around. So if you're missing a few ingredients – improvise! That's what makes it fun!*
- *Freshly brewed coffee (not instant) works best in this – if all you have is instant, then leave the coffee out and crumble in a stock cube instead.*
- *Haven't got stout? Any beer, will do, even lager. Sherry and white wine will do the trick as well.*
- *Use any hot seasoning mix you like – most supermarkets will have a shelf of various types.*

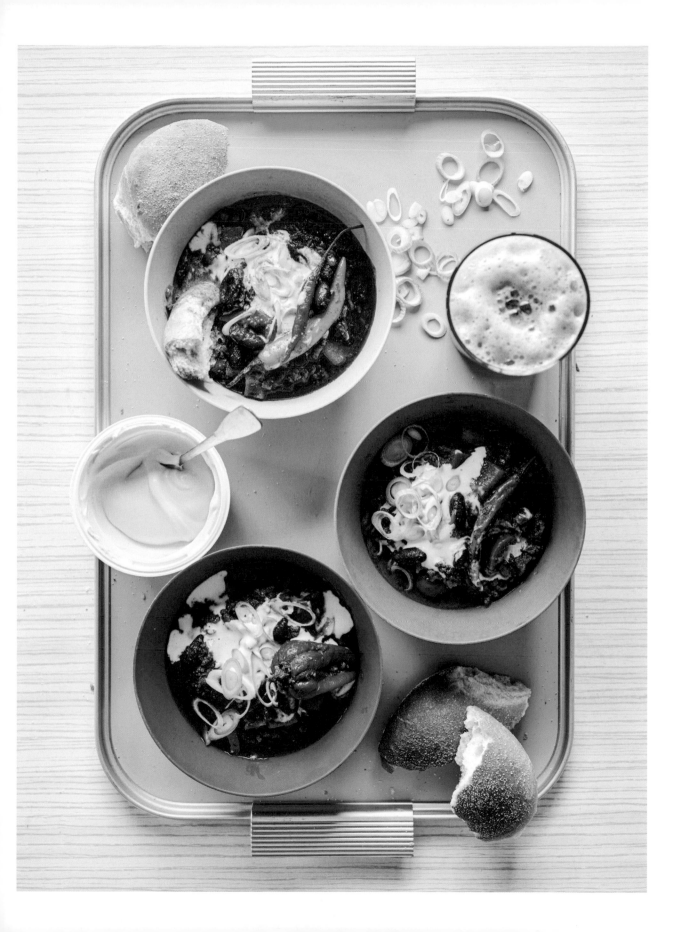

CHEESY MEATY PARCELS

Serves 4
469 calories

We came across this recipe while mincing around New York many moons ago. They used a fancy cheese whose name we didn't take note of, due to the fact we were hoovering up the wrap as quickly as we could before someone whose foot was wrapped in newspaper came over. We find that Cheddar makes a fine substitute.

This recipe looks incredibly simple, and honestly, we almost left it out of the book because it hardly needs any instruction at all. But this has been a go-to lunch many times over for us, so it has earned a place, nestled here among the dinners, for you all to enjoy. If you struggle with the idea of refried beans, you must work to get over it – they're delicious, low in fat and very filling.

Oh, and if you're concerned about buying steak for such a 'throwaway' meal, don't – we're not envisioning you tripping down to the shops and coming back with filet mignon – just some cheap beef steak will do just fine. All that extra chewing might give you a jaw like Desperate Dan, but you can take any jibes on your big, strong chin.

1 green and 1 red pepper, sliced
2 onions, finely sliced
2 small steaks (about 140g/5oz each), nowt fancy
2 tablespoons Worcestershire sauce
4 × 40g (1½ oz) wholemeal wraps
1 × 435g (15oz) tin of refried beans
shredded iceberg lettuce
100g (3½oz/1 cup) grated Cheddar cheese

Heat a frying pan over a medium-high heat and spray it with oil. Add the peppers and the onions and cook until softened.

Clear a space in the middle of the pan and chuck the steaks in. Depending on the thickness of your steaks, you want to cook them for about 3 minutes on each side – don't be moving them around, let them sear and char a little.

Place the steaks on a plate and add the Worcestershire sauce to the pan of onions and peppers. Cook them for a few minutes longer, and meanwhile slice your steaks – you don't need to do anything fancy here, just cut them however you want.

Assemble your wrap – add a good smear of refried beans, then the lettuce, then the steak, then the onions and peppers, followed by the cheese. Wrap, eat and enjoy.

Notes from Paul
- *This works well with chicken too, although we're all about the beef here at Chubby Towers.*
- *Feel free to add some corn tortilla chips into your wrap for a bit of crunch.*

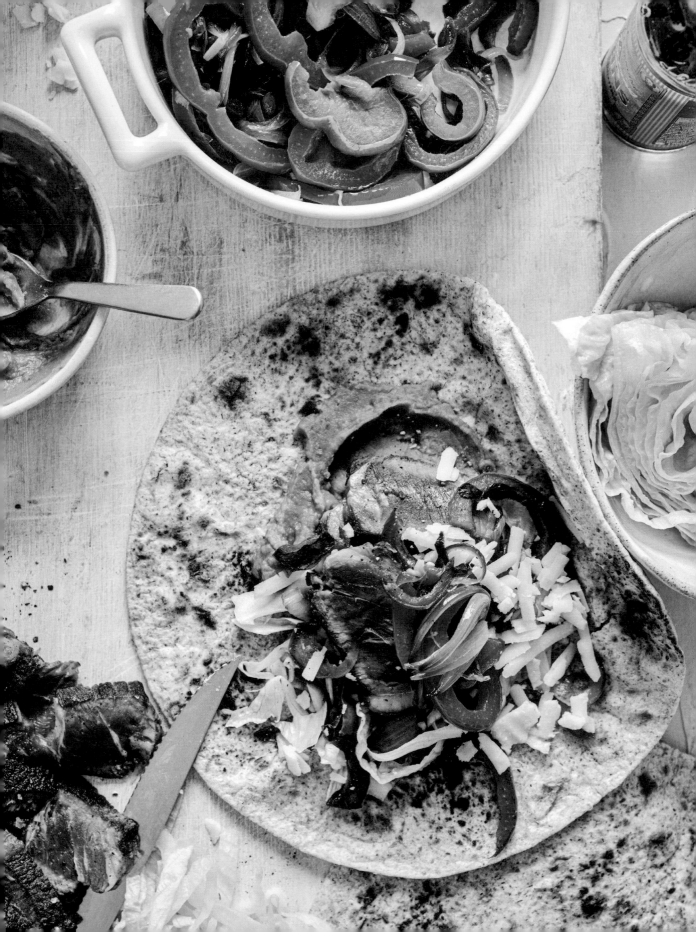

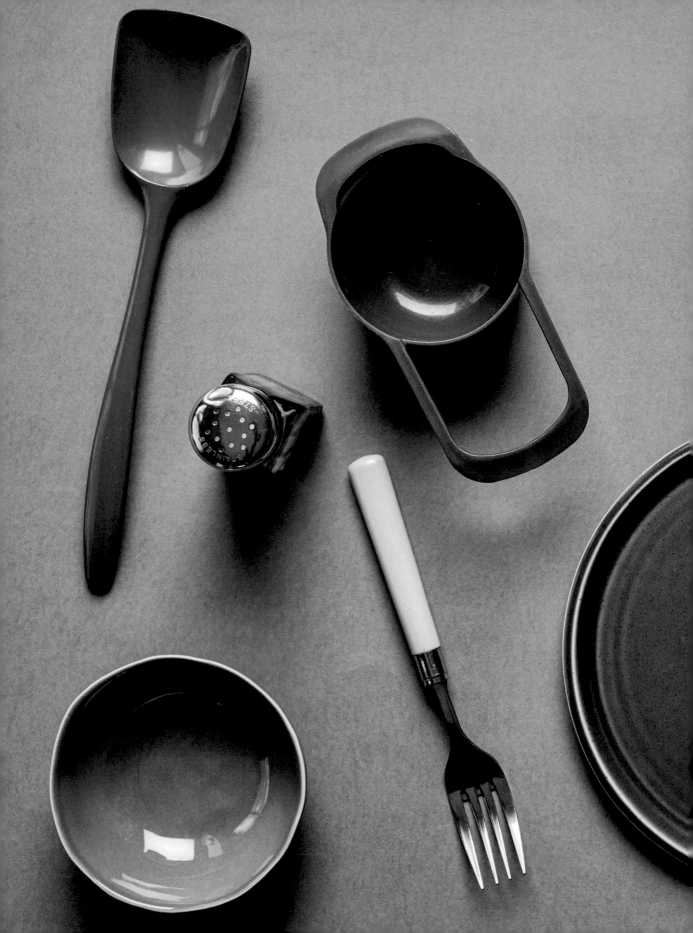

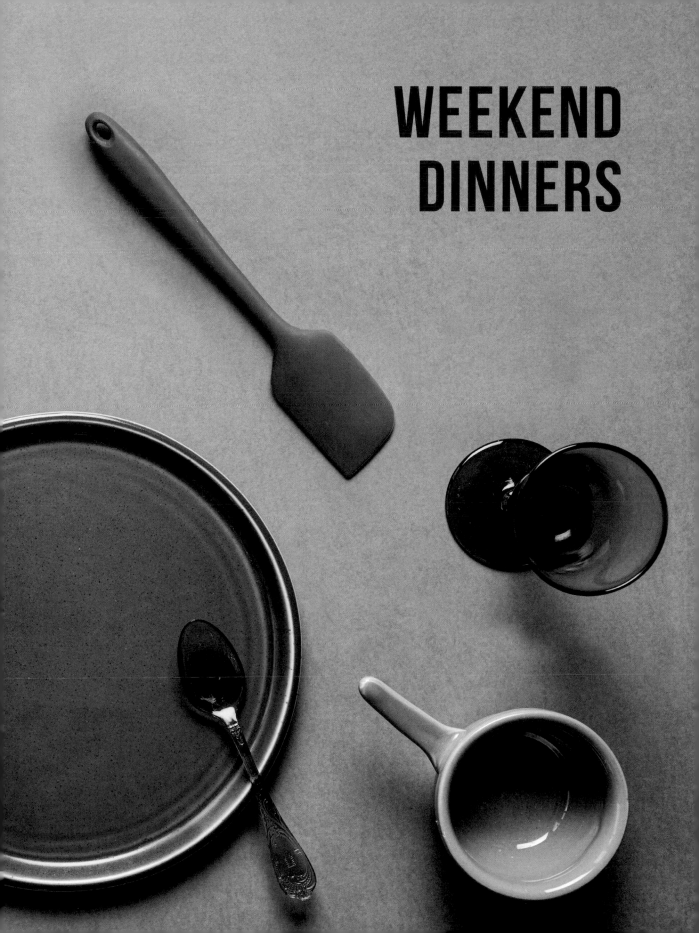

WEEKEND DINNERS

● ● ● ● ● ●

PAN-FRIED FIRECRACKER SALMON

Serves 4
250 calories

A few months into the weight-loss programme, we were drafted to take part in a boot camp. As the boot camp involved hour-long sessions of what they called HIIT – High Intensity Interval Training – we were getting home at 10pm feeling as though we had swam across an ocean. Knackered wasn't the word to describe us – after the first two sessions I actually collapsed to my knees in the front garden in full view of the neighbours.

We completed twelve weeks of it and actually, after the initial shock, it was bloody brilliant fun. Yes: fun. A particular highlight for me was the weekly boxing classes: there's something about being able to get all of that anger out into a trembling set of pads that really clicked with me. Paul had to ask me to pull back my punches a bit – I think he took it personally when I stitched his face onto the pads he was holding up.

Anyway, this salmon became a lifesaver. You can make the marinade in bulk and keep it in an airtight jar in the fridge, then on those days when you know it will be a struggle to blink let alone prepare tea, dig out some frozen salmon and get going.

2 cloves of garlic, crushed
¼ teaspoon ground ginger
¼ teaspoon hot chilli powder
1 tablespoon soy sauce
3 teaspoons sriracha
1 teaspoon honey
½ teaspoon smoked paprika
4 salmon fillets, around 120g (4oz) each

Mix all the ingredients apart from the salmon together in a bowl to make the marinade.

Put the salmon into a large sandwich bag and pour in the marinade, turning gently to ensure the fish is well coated. Leave to marinate for a couple of hours in the fridge.

Heat a large frying pan over a medium heat. Place the salmon in the pan, spoon over any excess marinade and cook on each side for 3 minutes.

Notes from Paul

- *We have these with boiled new potatoes, a rocket salad and a loo roll cooling in the fridge.*
- *Salmon isn't tricky to cook – after a few minutes, take a look at the thickest part of your fillet – you want it almost white, with just a hint of pink in the middle*

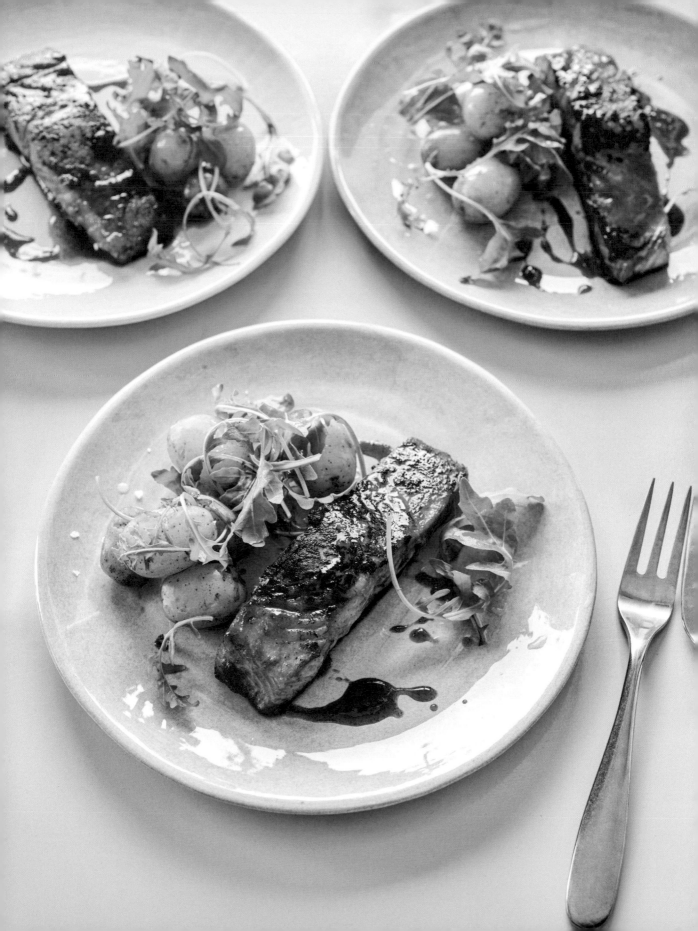

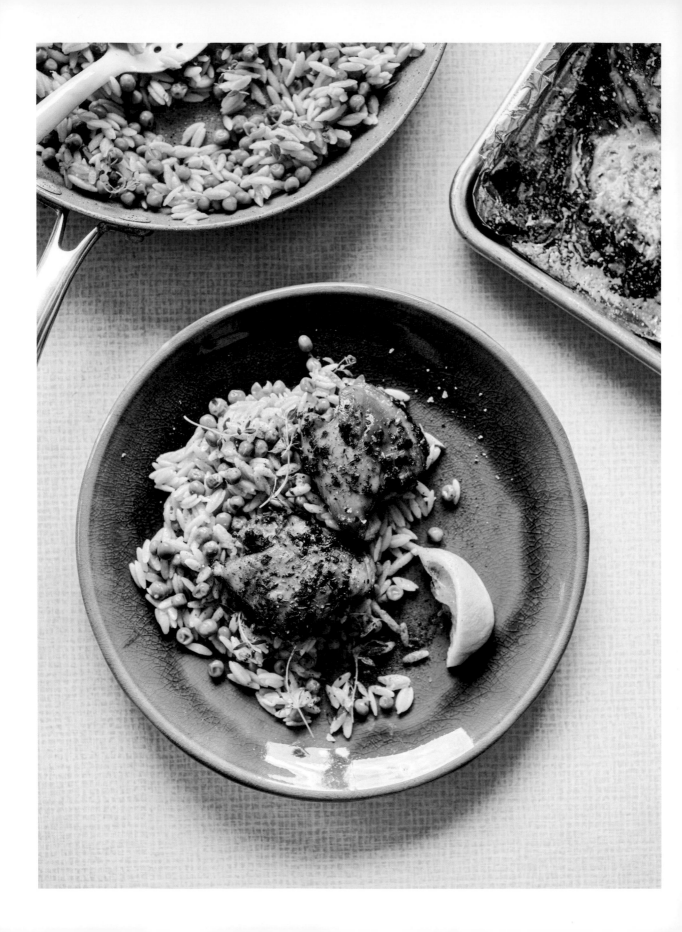

LEMON CHICKEN WITH ORZO

Serves 4
495 calories

This dish is one of those meals you can throw together of an evening and spend a few absent-minded minutes stirring while looking moonily at your handsome neighbour over the road. Orzo is easy to find in supermarkets, though not if you're me: I spent a good half-hour swearing at the shelves and sweating before I realized that orzo isn't rice but pasta – some kindly soul in winceyette shuffled me down the aisle a bit and I've never looked back. If you do struggle, though, don't hesitate to swap it out for whatever tiny pasta you can find. We shan't judge.

We get asked a lot via the blog what we make when we just 'can't be bothered', and honestly, that feeling occurs so much more often than you might think. Finding recipes and trying new things will always be exciting, but sometimes you just need a meal you know will work, that tastes good and requires minimal effort. This is one of those.

If you have any leftover orzo and chicken, shred the chicken down, mix with the leftover orzo and leave to dry out a little in the fridge overnight. Then the next day, form it into 'burgers' and gently fry them – absolutely fantastic with some sour cream.

4 cloves of garlic, crushed
2 teaspoons onion granules
2 teaspoons dried mixed herbs
1 teaspoon freshly ground black pepper
½ teaspoon paprika
6 boneless chicken thighs
300g (10½oz/1½ cups) orzo
½ teaspoon dried thyme
750ml (1¼ pints/3 cups) chicken stock
zest and juice of 1 lemon
150g (5½oz/1 cup) peas, cooked and drained (see note)

Preheat the oven to 200°C fan/425°F/gas mark 7 and line a large baking tray with tin foil.

Mix together half the crushed garlic cloves, the onion granules, mixed herbs, black pepper and paprika, and rub this mix over the chicken thighs. Place on the lined baking tray and cook in the oven for 40 minutes.

Meanwhile, heat a large pan over a medium heat and spray with a bit of oil. Add the orzo and cook for 45–60 seconds, stirring continuously. Add the rest of the crushed garlic cloves to the pan with the thyme and stir well, then stir in the chicken stock a little at a time.

Bring to the boil, then cover and reduce to a simmer for about 8–10 minutes, until the orzo is cooked.

Remove the lid, add the lemon zest, juice and peas, and stir well.

Serve the chicken with the orzo.

Notes from Paul
- You can use chicken breasts instead of thighs if you prefer.
- Frozen peas will work fine in this – just whack them in the microwave for 30 seconds or so to thaw them a bit before chucking them in.
- Orzo is pasta, but looks like rice – you'll find it in most supermarkets.

• • • • • •

CHICKEN ACHARI

Serves 4
312 calories

1 teaspoon mustard seeds
1 teaspoon fennel seeds
1 teaspoon cumin seeds
2 red chillies
1 onion, finely sliced
3cm (1½ inches) ginger, peeled
    and crushed
4 cloves of garlic, crushed
1½ tablespoons tomato purée
½ teaspoon ground turmeric
½ teaspoon onion powder
2 teaspoons hot chilli powder
750g (1½lb) boneless, skinless
    chicken thighs
100g (3½oz/½ cup) yoghurt
chopped fresh coriander,
    to serve

For years I thwarted any attempt to use chicken thighs; recipe after recipe would be swiped-left because I liked an uncomplicated bite and the thought of gristle and bone touching my teeth was an absolute no-no. I thought I was alone with my fussiness until I met Paul, who confirmed he also had a similar phobia.

However, this recipe (sort of) won us round to chicken thighs because, after years of totally disregarding them, we noticed that you can now buy boneless thighs. Well, bugger me: what a difference in taste. A breast is fine for most things, but chicken thighs absolutely lend themselves to a dish like this – the more 'meaty' flavour works well with the spices and really lifts the dish. Don't be afraid!

Heat a large pan over a medium heat and spray with some oil. Add the mustard, fennel and cumin seeds and fry for about a minute until they start to sizzle, then add the chillies to the pan, whole.

Add the sliced onion and fry until it is just turning golden and has softened. Add the ginger and garlic and stir well. Stir in the tomato purée, turmeric, onion powder and chilli powder and cook for a few more minutes, then add the chicken to the pan and stir gently until well coated.

Pour in 100ml (3½fl oz/½ cup) of water and bring to the boil, then cover the pan and reduce to a simmer over a low heat. Cook for 20 minutes, stirring occasionally, then remove from the heat and add the yoghurt, stirring gently.

Keep stirring now and again for another 5 minutes or so, then serve, sprinkled with chopped coriander.

Notes from Paul
- *Don't be tempted to use fat-free or low-fat yoghurt for this – IT WILL SPLIT! You'll need the full-fat stuff, but there's not a lot per person so don't worry too much about the calories – it'll be worth it, I promise.*
- *If you're not a fan of food being too hot, feel free to reduce the amount of chilli powder or the number of chillies to something you're more comfortable with.*
- *Chicken breasts would work well in this too – just cut them in half before you put them in.*

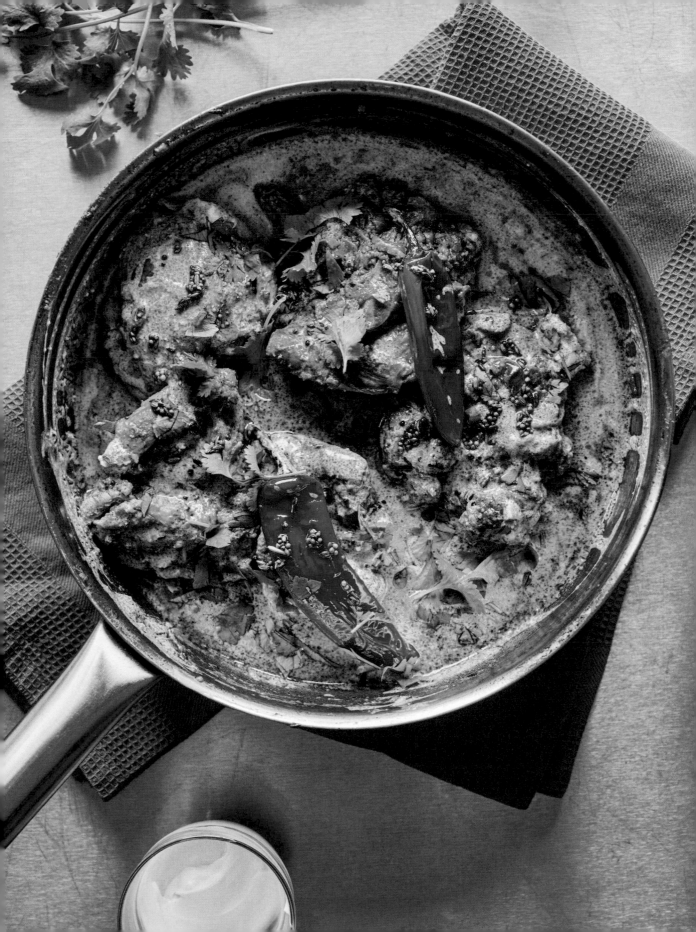

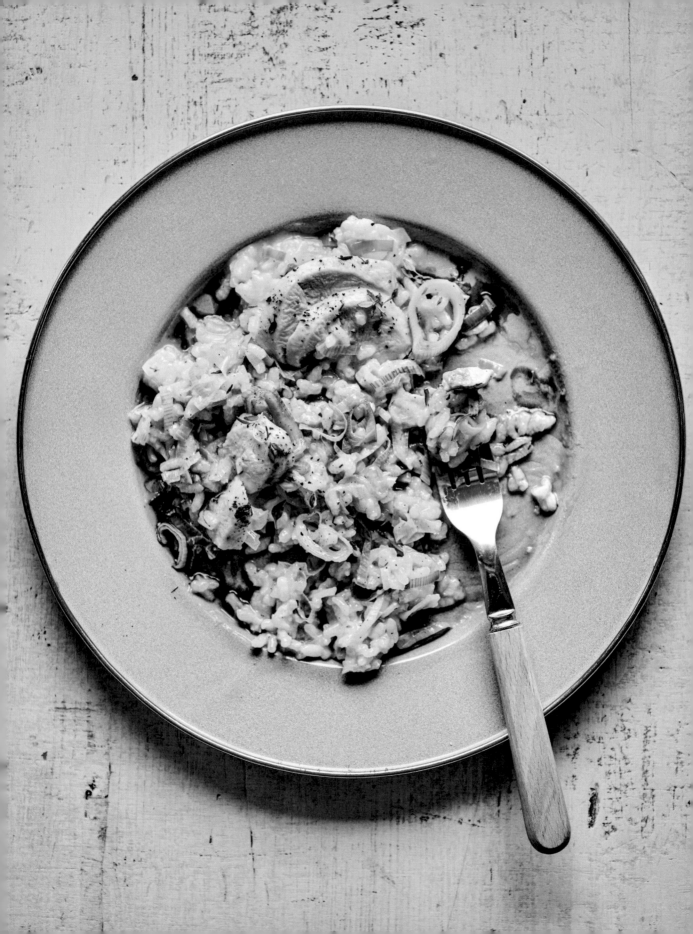

• • • • • •

SUNSHINE RISOTTO

Serves 4
487 calories

We're calling this 'sunshine risotto' because frankly, chicken and thyme – though delicious – doesn't lend itself to an exciting recipe title. It's a pale yellow, so it was either 'sunshine risotto' or 'a bowl full of jaundice'. That's marketing at work right there. But it's a happy little dish, and that rather reflects well on your author.

See, I'm not one for staring at my shoes and feeling sorry for myself. Lord knows I used to be – a scatty remark or a pointed glance would send me into a tailspin that many tubs of ice cream and tears would barely touch. I don't want to dwell, but this is an important point. When you're overweight, you make your world smaller in so many ways. Going to the cinema becomes an exercise in choosing the right seat so you're not having to thrust your arse in someone's face as you struggle past them. Theme parks are a bust because what if you don't fit in the rides? Even going to a restaurant becomes a chore: people looking at you while you eat, judging your choices, trying not to giggle as your lips smack together.

You have two choices here: carry on feeling sorry for yourself, or take my approach of not giving a toss anymore. I use the recollection exercise – did you go to the supermarket yesterday? Can you remember a single person you saw? What they were wearing? Of course you can't, unless a hottie walked past. And see, this is why you shouldn't worry: no one will remember you either. And mind, that's not a criticism of you, I hasten to add, but rather a call as to why you shouldn't care what strangers think. That's the me approach, and it's a much, much better way to live.

1 leek, finely sliced
60ml (2fl oz/¼ cup) balsamic
　　vinegar
350g (12½oz/1¾ cups) Arborio
　　rice
60ml (2fl oz/¼ cup) white wine
2 skinless, boneless chicken
　　breasts, cooked and diced
1.6 litres (2¾ pints/6 cups)
　　chicken stock
2 teaspoons dried thyme

Heat a medium-sized saucepan over a medium heat and spray with some oil. Add the leeks and cook for 15–20 minutes, until they are a golden brown colour. Remove from the heat and stir in the balsamic vinegar, then set aside.

Heat a large frying pan over a medium heat, spray with some oil and add the rice. Let the rice heat for about 1–2 minutes, then add the wine, stirring well. Reduce the heat and stir in the chicken, then add the stock slowly, a ladleful at a time, stirring continuously until it's all been absorbed – which will take about 15–20 minutes.

Stir in the leeks and thyme, then cook for another minute or 2 and serve.

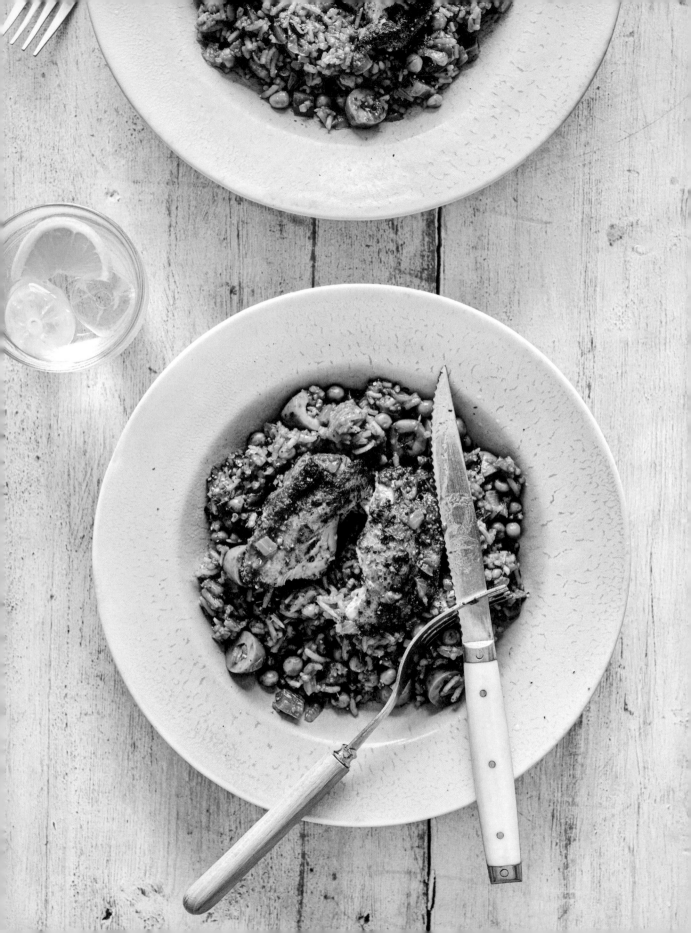

● ● ● ○ ● ●

ARROZ CON POLLO

Serves 4
496 calories

Arroz con pollo might sound like something you'd see a nurse about behind a closed curtain, but we can assure you that it's actually a very delicious, traditional dish that, although the list of ingredients seems long and daunting, is a doddle to pull together. The chicken takes a leisurely marinade in all the spices, the pan is used for everything else, and you'll be serving this up to rapturous applause and happy tears in no time at all.

This recipe is actually one of Paul's rare finds. He's a fan of finding an excuse to use every single spice we have in the cupboard – I'm sure if we look hard enough beyond the panko graveyard, Geri Halliwell will come trotting out in a Union Jack dress. Or me, I've certainly got the bust.

700g (1lb 9oz) skinless, boneless
  chicken thighs

For the seasoning
1 teaspoon each of ground cumin
  and paprika
½ teaspoon each of cayenne
  pepper, hot chilli powder,
  onion granules, garlic
  granules, salt and freshly
  ground black pepper
¼ teaspoon ground coriander

For the rice
3 cloves of garlic, crushed
1 large onion, finely diced
1 green pepper, finely diced
½ handful of fresh coriander
  leaves, chopped
a few jalapeño slices (from a jar),
  chopped
¼ teaspoon each of ground
  coriander, ground cumin,
  ground turmeric, garlic
  granules, dried oregano, salt
  and freshly ground black
  pepper
250g (9oz/1 cup) passata
100g (3½oz/¾ cup) frozen peas
16 pitted green olives, halved
180g (6¼oz/1 cup) white rice

Place the chicken thighs in a bowl.

Mix together all the seasoning ingredients and sprinkle over the chicken. Stir well, then cover the bowl with cling film and leave to marinate for at least 30 minutes.

Heat a large pan over a medium-high heat and spray generously with oil. Add the chicken and cook for 4–5 minutes on each side, then remove from the pan on to a plate.

Add the garlic, onion, green pepper, coriander leaves and jalapeños to the pan and fry for 2 minutes, stirring constantly, then reduce the heat to medium and add the ground coriander, cumin, turmeric, garlic granules, oregano, salt and pepper. Cook for another 30 seconds.

Add the passata, peas, olives and 300ml (10fl oz/1¼ cups) of water to the pan and stir well. Add the rice and stir again, then reduce the heat to low and place the chicken thighs on top of the rice mixture.

Cover with a lid and simmer for 20–25 minutes.

Serve in big warmed bowls.

WE'LL LET YOU IN ON A SECRET — JERK SEASONING FROM THE SUPERMARKETS WILL GET YOU THE SAME RESULT FOR THE CHICKEN.

ULTIMATE COMFORT CHICKEN SOUP

Serves 4
362 calories

You may think we're over-selling this recipe a little, given there's no cream or butter in there to grease it along, but honestly, it's one of the nicest chicken soup recipes we have ever made. Starting off with skimmed milk keeps everything nice and light, but it doesn't taste like you have skimped on the calories. Just the thing if you're feeling a little under the weather, with the added bonus of consisting of ingredients you will likely find rattling around in your cupboards.

Neither of us copes well with being ill – Paul is very much a 'mention he is ill every twenty minutes but then do nothing about it' sort of guy, whereas I'm firmly of the belief that every slight twinge and ache is a sign that I should get my affairs in order and book the crematorium.

The recipe, then – it makes more than enough for four big hearty bowls.

1 litre (1¾ pints/4 cups) skimmed milk, or semi-skimmed if you're feeling like a decadent hussy
2 large skinless, boneless chicken breasts
2 tablespoons cornflour
1 celery stalk, finely chopped
300g (10½oz/2 cups) frozen veg mix
100g (3½oz/1½ cups) button mushrooms, sliced
1 onion, chopped
2 chicken stock cubes
a pinch of dried thyme
a pinch of freshly ground black pepper
2 medium potatoes, peeled and cut into tiny cubes

Poach the chicken by bringing the milk up to simmering point, popping the chicken in and letting it bubble away for 15 minutes. Remove the chicken from the pan and pop it on to a plate.

Mix the cornflour with 100ml (3½fl oz/½ cup) of cold water and set aside.

Reheat the milk with 750ml (1¼ pints/3 cups) of water and bring slowly to the boil. Add the celery, veg mix, mushrooms and onion, along with the crumbled stock cubes, thyme and black pepper. Bring to the boil, then cover and leave to simmer for around 25 minutes.

Add the potato cubes and keep cooking for another 5 minutes.

Use 2 forks to shred your chicken and tip it into the pan.

Dribble the cornflour mix into the soup, making sure to whisk thoroughly as you go, otherwise: ructions.

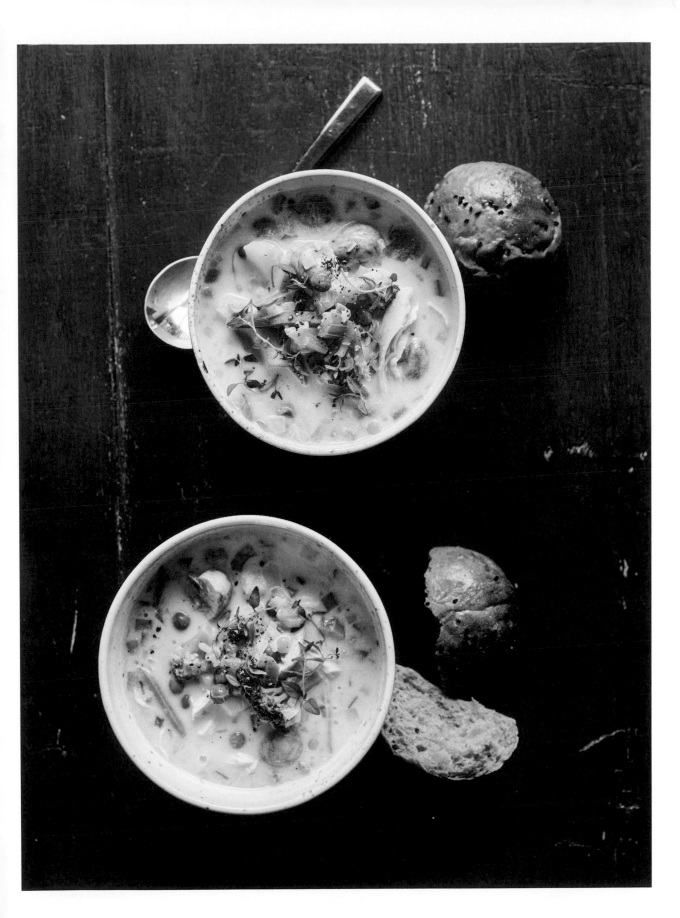

OH THE HUMANITY CHICKEN

Serves 4
479 calories

1 tablespoon dried mixed herbs
1 tablespoon dried rosemary
1 teaspoon salt
1 teaspoon freshly ground black
    pepper
2 teaspoons onion granules
2 teaspoons garlic granules
2 teaspoons paprika
3 tablespoons olive oil
1 × 440ml (15½fl oz) can of
    Guinness
1 large chicken (ours was
    1.5kg/3lb)

Goodness me, what to say about a recipe where the photo is a chicken with a can of beer stuck up its rear end?

While Paul and I were writing this book, we were asked to record a podcast where we talked about our favourite recipes. I mentioned this recipe where you shove a can of beer somewhere indecent so the beer flavour comes through from the inside and makes things moist and delicious. Paul immediately jumped in to say the beer can goes down the throat.

I mean, what chicken has he seen that can accommodate a can of Guinness in its throat? This turned into a ten-minute argument, which only ended when the poor chap monitoring the sound levels came bursting in to tell us to get a move on and, anyway, it definitely isn't the bloody neck. You can actually hear the smugness in my voice for a good fifteen minutes after.

If you will struggle to get a chicken standing up in the oven or you don't want use the beer, that's absolutely fine. The rub is one of our favourites and you can absolutely get away with using a little more oil and doing this as a normal roast. But we're all about the theatre at Chubby Towers.

Preheat the oven to 220°C fan/475°F/gas mark 9, removing all the oven shelves. Mix the herbs, seasoning and spices with the oil and rub into the skin of the chicken.

Pour out 100ml (3½fl oz/½ cup) of the beer into a roasting tin. Put the open, upright can containing the rest of the beer into the roasting tin and carefully squat the chicken over the top, pushing down until the chicken is able to stand up.

Roast in the oven for around 1 hour and 20 minutes, or until golden and at the right temperature when tested with a meat thermometer (see note). Serve with potato wedges or a simple salad.

Notes from Paul
- *Make sure the chicken is big enough to, ahem, 'accommodate' the can, though not too big that it might topple over – if you're struggling, the traditional recipe suggests folding the legs down to act as stabilizers.*
- *Your chicken is cooked when the juices run clear, but honestly, please get a meat thermometer. Stick it into the part of the chicken where the thighs and drumsticks meet – you want a minimum of 75°C/167°F.*
- *Be careful when removing the chicken – the can will be VERY hot, and the chicken will be distraught if you don't call her afterwards.*
- *Don't bloody drink the beer in the can, whatever you do; however, you can certainly make a fantastic gravy from the juices in the roasting pan – sieve in a little cornflour, stir in some Worcestershire sauce and serve.*

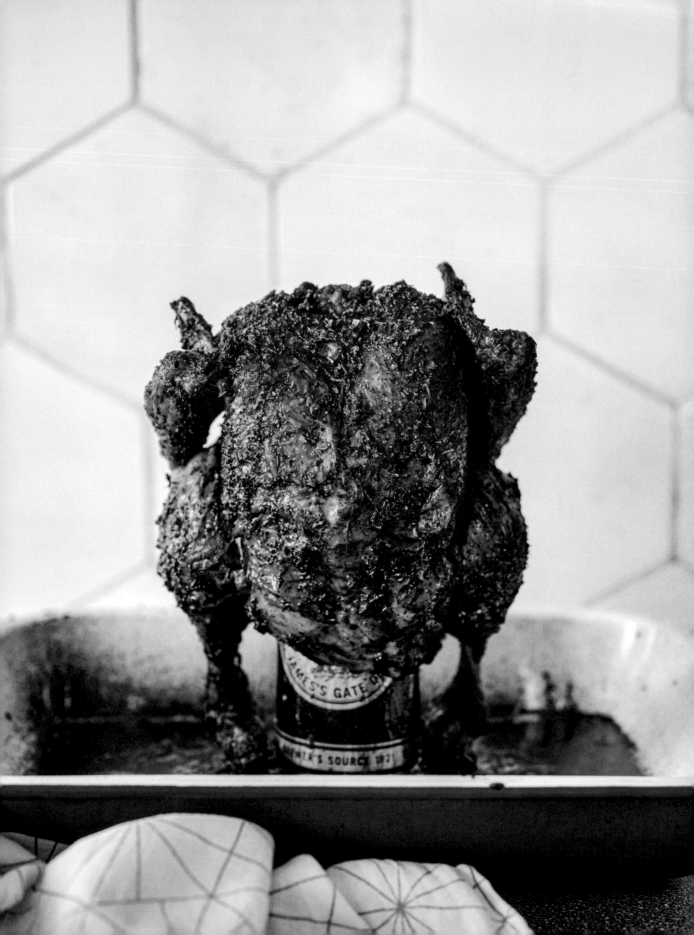

SUPER TASTY TURKEY MEATBALLS

Serves 4
327 calories

Turkey gets quite the bum rap in cooking circles, doesn't it? But my favourite cooking circle, Paul, swears by it. It can be a smidge dry, certainly, but mix it with the right ingredients, throw it in a curry or, in this case, tasty meatballs, and you're onto a winner. A note of caution though: turkey mince does have rather the tendency to be a little 'wet' – if you find this is the case, feel free to up the amount of breadcrumbs.

There's a recipe on our blog for basil and turkey mince served on a bed of glass noodles which has been filed away in the 'never republish' category. Not because it's a failed recipe, but because goodness me, the photography is shocking. We never aimed to be one of those blogs where the food photography takes longer than cooking the actual dish. What you see in the photos is one of maybe four photos I've managed to snap before Paul starts picking at the plate with his sausage-fingers. If it happens to look halfway decent, then it's nothing more than luck, trust me.

I'm sure some studious sort would tell us that if we posed the food just so, we'd get all sorts of excited fans. But listen: we want to appeal to those folks who just want to eat. People like us – so here we are!

500g (1lb 2oz) turkey mince
30g (1oz/1 cup) fresh sage leaves, chopped
1 egg
60g (2¼oz/¾ cup) grated Parmesan cheese
30g (1oz/⅓ cup) breadcrumbs
6 bacon medallions, diced into small cubes
275g (9¾oz) cherry tomatoes
1 red onion, finely diced
1 teaspoon crushed chilli flakes
6 cloves of garlic, crushed
1.25 litres (2¼ pints/5 cups) chicken stock
250g (9oz) swede and carrot mix (see note)
60ml (2fl oz/¼ cup) semi-skimmed milk

Put the turkey mince, sage, egg, Parmesan and breadcrumbs into a bowl and mix together with your hands. Divide the mixture into about 20 portions, roll them into meatballs, and set them aside.

Spray a large saucepan with oil and place over a medium heat. Add the bacon and cook until crispy, then remove it from the pan with a spoon.

Increase the heat to medium-high and add the cherry tomatoes. Cook for about 5–6 minutes, until they begin to blister, stirring regularly. Spray a little more oil into the pan and add the onion, chilli flakes and garlic. Cook, stirring, for 1–2 minutes.

Pour the stock into the pan and bring to the boil. Cook for 5–6 minutes, then add the bacon and reduce the heat to a simmer. Add the swede and carrot mix to the pan and return to a simmer.

Carefully drop the meatballs into the liquid in a single layer. Bring back to a simmer, then cover the pan and cook for about 10 minutes, until the meatballs have cooked through. Stir in the milk and serve.

Note from Paul
We use the prepared bags of diced swede and carrots, but if there's something else you prefer, feel free to use that instead. Potatoes would work well too – just be sure to either parboil them a bit first or chop them into small pieces to make sure they cook through.

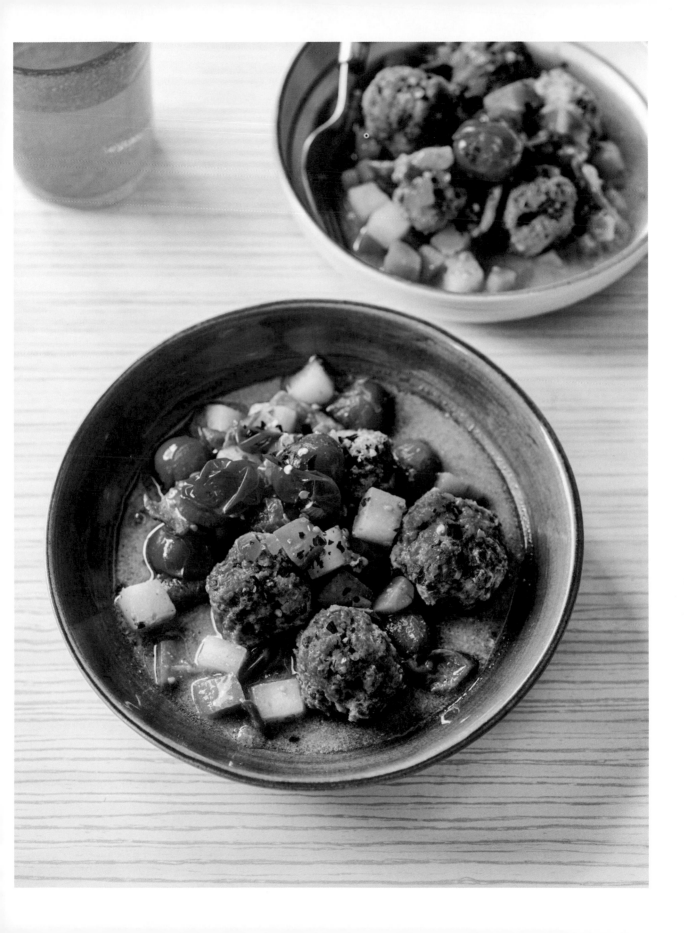

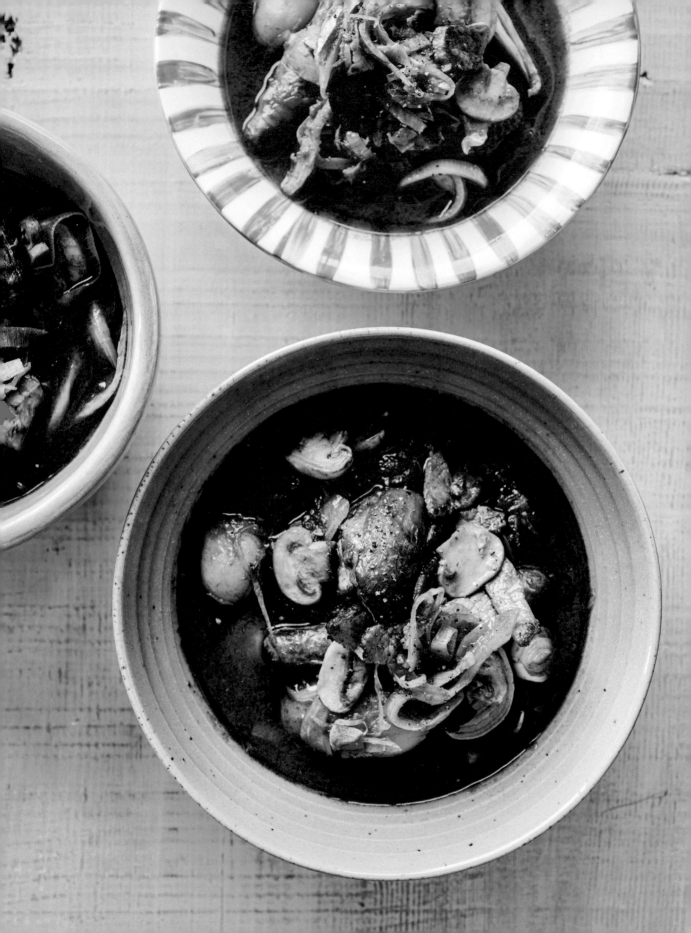

• • • • • •

POLISH STEW

Serves 4
494 calories

2 red peppers
4 tomatoes
400g (14oz) skinless, boneless
    chicken thighs
4 bacon medallions, diced
1 onion, diced
300g (10½oz/4½ cups) button
    mushrooms, sliced
4 low-fat pork sausages
1 bulb of fennel, thinly sliced
1 leek, thinly sliced
5 cloves of garlic, sliced
3 tablespoons paprika
1 × 540g (1lb 3oz) tin of new
    potatoes, drained
250ml (9fl oz/1 cup) red wine
1 litre (1¾ pints/4 cups) chicken
    stock
600g (1lb 5oz) sauerkraut

This is a recipe that always gets trotted out towards Christmas, because it feels like one of those meals that lends itself to a cold, stormy evening. When you've been married as long as we have been, every evening is cold and stormy, but we make do.

You mustn't be afraid of sauerkraut, by the way. Yes, you open the jar and it smells like something broke wind and died in the kitchen, but it's bloody lovely stuff. The vinegar-and-farts smell evaporates off and leaves you with a lovely thick stew.

Put the red peppers (whole) under a high grill and cook for 5–6 minutes, turning occasionally, until the skins are blistered and blackened. Transfer to a plate and set aside to cool for 5–10 minutes.

Slice off the stems of the peppers and remove the seeds, then place the peppers in a food processor with the tomatoes and blitz until smooth.

Spray a large casserole dish with a little oil and place over a medium-high heat. Add the chicken and cook until browned, about 5 minutes per side, then transfer to a plate.

Add the bacon to the same dish and cook for a few minutes, then add the onion and mushrooms and cook until the onion is starting to turn brown. Add the sausages, fennel, leek, garlic and paprika and cook for about 7–8 minutes, stirring occasionally.

Return the chicken to the dish along with the new potatoes, wine and 200ml (7fl oz/¾ cup) of stock, and bring to the boil. Add the pepper and tomato mixture, along with the sauerkraut and the rest of the stock, simmer for about 45 minutes, then serve.

Note from Paul
Chicken thighs give the best flavour, but chicken breasts will work too.

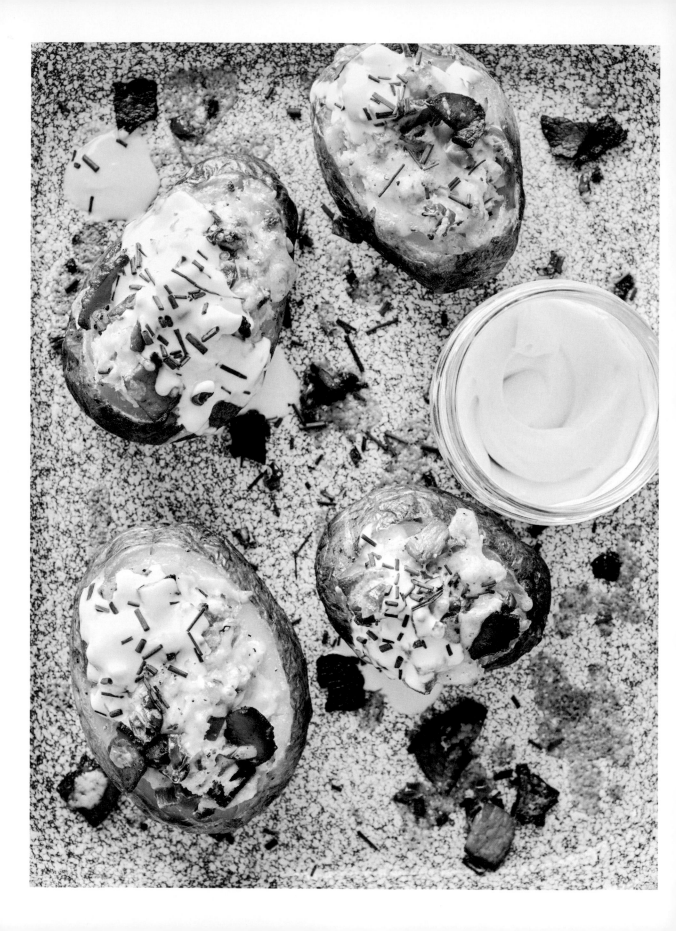

CHILLI CHEESE JACKET POTATOES

Serves 4
500 calories

Can you beat the humble jacket potato for a quick lunch? Rolled in a little olive oil, sprinkled with sea salt and then baked slowly for as long as you can get away with. I will happily die on the hill of the best 'takeaway', that being those potatoes that you get in museum cafes which have been baking since the Boer War in those specialized potato ovens. Crunchy on the outside, absolute mush in the middle, covered with beans and that plastic orange shredded cheese that has no sooner come from a cow than I have.

Paul just confessed to me his guilty jacket potato secret, which has to be the most boring revelation I've ever heard, but let's hear him out. Turns out that when he first started in the halls of residence at Cambridge (there must have been one hell of an admin mix-up there, just saying) he had absolutely bot-all money and lived on potatoes for the first week. One evening, somewhat 'tired and emotional', he threw a potato in the oven and then 'went to rest his eyes'. Woke to find the fire alarm blaring and the kitchen full of smoke. So panicked was he that he'd almost torched the place in the search of carbs, he raced into the kitchen, grabbed the potato and stole it away on top of his wardrobe where almost doubtless, given his hands-off approach to cleaning, it remains even now.

These jacket potatoes, topped as they are with a rich chilli and baked twice, are a treat. However, savvy readers will use any leftover chilli from the five-alarm chilli (see page 138) to really speed up this dish.

4 medium baking potatoes
200g (7oz) bacon medallions, diced
160g (5¾oz/1½ cups) reduced-fat Cheddar cheese, grated
150g (5½oz/¾ cup) light soft cheese
½ teaspoon garlic granules
½ teaspoon onion granules
2 teaspoons sriracha
3 green chillies, deseeded and finely diced
½ teaspoon freshly ground black pepper
4 tablespoons reduced-fat crème fraîche, to serve
fresh chives, chopped, to serve

Preheat the oven to 180°C fan/400°F/gas mark 6.

Prick the potatoes all over with a fork, rub them with a little olive oil, and bake in the oven for 70 minutes. Remove them from the oven and leave for 10 minutes to cool.

Meanwhile, heat a small frying pan over a high heat and add the bacon. Stir it round the pan until crisp, then remove from the heat.

Slice the top quarter off each potato and scoop the soft insides into a bowl. Mix in the Cheddar, soft cheese, garlic and onion granules, bacon, sriracha, chillies and black pepper, reserving a tablespoon each of the bacon, Cheddar and chillies.

Spoon the potato mix back into the potatoes and top each one with the reserved ingredients. Bake in the oven for a further 15 minutes, then remove from the oven and top with a tablespoon of crème fraîche and a sprinkling of chives.

Note from Paul
Keep any leftover mixture in the fridge to shovel in your gob every time you make a brew.

• • • • • •

SLOW COOKER MEATBALL SOUP

Serves 4
417 calories

For years, our slow cooker languished in the cupboard of sin in the kitchen, hidden between the spiralizer we never used, the sandwich toaster we never cleaned and all the lovely tchotchkes and tat we had bought from charity shops with the sole intention of using them for decoration on the blog. Open that cupboard door and everything tumbles out like the worst episode of The Generation Game you've ever seen.

The slow cooker was ignored for a silly reason, though – I was terrified of leaving something switched on all day while we were at work. Paul mocks me when I leave the house, as I turn everything off and pull out the plugs as though electricity and fire are going to come pouring from the sockets, but know this: I once saw a faulty plug burn down a lovely semi-detached on 999 back in the nineties and frankly, if you can't trust Michael Buerk, who can you trust?

It took Paul going over my head – a difficult feat when I'm six foot two to his three foot barely – to overcome this phobia. He waited until I had left early for work and set a beer and barley stew to cook through the day. I only realized what he had done when I came home and noticed the house smelling like my nana's kitchen. I was converted there and then, to rapturous and extensive applause.

Now, we're huge fans of the slow cooker here at Chubby Towers and use it for all manner of exciting dishes, from slow-cooked pork to slow-cooked beef, and even slow-cooked chicken. I know! But actually, this slow-cooked meatball dish is a treat and we encourage you to give it a whirl.

250g (9oz) lean pork mince
2 chicken stock cubes
1 onion, finely chopped
2 celery stalks, finely chopped
2 carrots, finely chopped
2 × 400g (14oz) tins of chopped
   tomatoes
3 tablespoons tomato purée
2 teaspoons mixed herbs
500g (1lb 2oz) gnocchi
30g (1oz/¼ cup) Parmesan
   cheese,
   to serve
a few leaves of fresh basil,
   to serve

Divide the pork mince into 12 portions and roll them into meatballs.

Dissolve the stock cubes in 600ml (20fl oz/2½ cups) of boiling water.

Chuck everything except for the gnocchi, Parmesan and basil into the slow cooker and cook on low for 4 hours.

Add the gnocchi to the slow cooker and cook for another hour.

If you don't have a slow cooker, reduce the amount of water to 400ml (14fl oz/1¾ cups) and cook in a lidded casserole dish in the oven at 180°C fan/400°F/gas mark 6 for 20–25 minutes.

Serve in bowls, grate over the Parmesan and sprinkle with the basil.

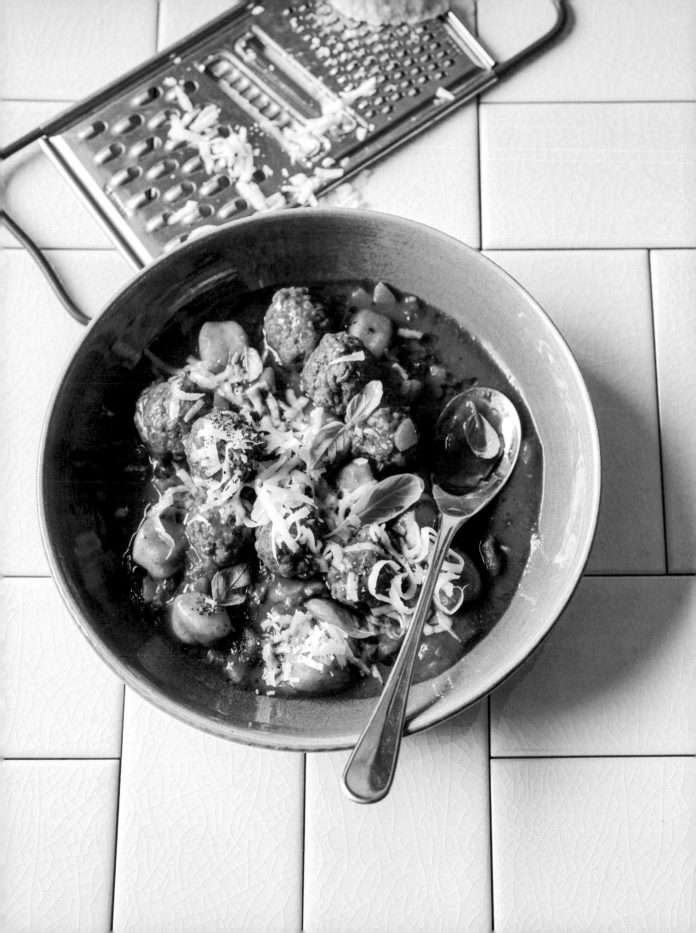

• • • • • •

OUR FIRST DATE FANCY SPAGHETTI SAUCE

Serves 4
453 calories

When we first started 'dating', Paul excitedly decided to cook a meal for me. Picture this: two young, handsome men circling around one another, trying to impress each other and hiding all of our faults and weaknesses. I imagined some delicious four-course dinner, each serving cementing his love for me more and more. I had a shave, popped on my best shirt (which is any shirt that doesn't have egg dropped down the front), and took a seat at the table, eager for some culinary delights.

He served up a plate of badly mashed potato and mince. The mince was grey as a dead toe and entirely lacking in gravy, flavour, onion, garlic – anything that would have made it exciting. It was simply mince. Never before has someone fallen so quickly in my estimation, and it was all I could do not to make an excuse to nip back home (which would have been a feat – Portsmouth to Newcastle is quite a trek). I smiled wanly and choked back this dismal repast with tears in my eyes. Paul took this as validation and made to get me a second portion, to which I had to feign fullness and try to distract him with the offer of some youthful, energetic sex.

This recipe isn't his famous grey-mince-and-mash spread, but rather the first meal I cooked for him – you'll note that it's far more fancy. We cook this a lot even now, because it's easy, low in fat and infinitely customizable. It won Paul's heart, after all. Give it a go, though I make no apology if a portly gentleman appears at your side and never leaves.

3 large shallots, finely chopped
200g (7oz) smoked bacon lardons
1 clove of garlic, crushed
1 × 400g (14oz) tin of cherry tomatoes (or use plum tomatoes if you're not as fancy)
250g (9oz/1 cup) passata
100g (3½oz/¾ cup) pitted black olives, chopped
285g (10oz) artichoke hearts in oil, drained and finely chopped
200g (7oz) dried spaghetti (or as much spaghetti as you feel you need to fill yourself)
1 large bag of spinach (about 100g/3½oz)

Gently cook the shallots and bacon together in a pan until the bacon is cooked through.

Add the garlic and cook for a minute or 2, then add the tinned tomatoes, passata, olives and artichoke hearts and allow to bubble for a good 30 minutes, until everything has reduced nicely.

Towards the end of the bubbling, cook your spaghetti according to the packet instructions. As soon as you've drained the spaghetti, tip it back into the pan and add the spinach so the leaves wilt in the heat of the pasta.

Serve with the tomato sauce atop the spaghetti and spinach, or mix everything together.

Notes from Paul
- *Don't salt the spaghetti water – the saltiness of the bacon will be enough, I promise.*
- *If you're not covering this with as much cheese as you can, are you even living?*

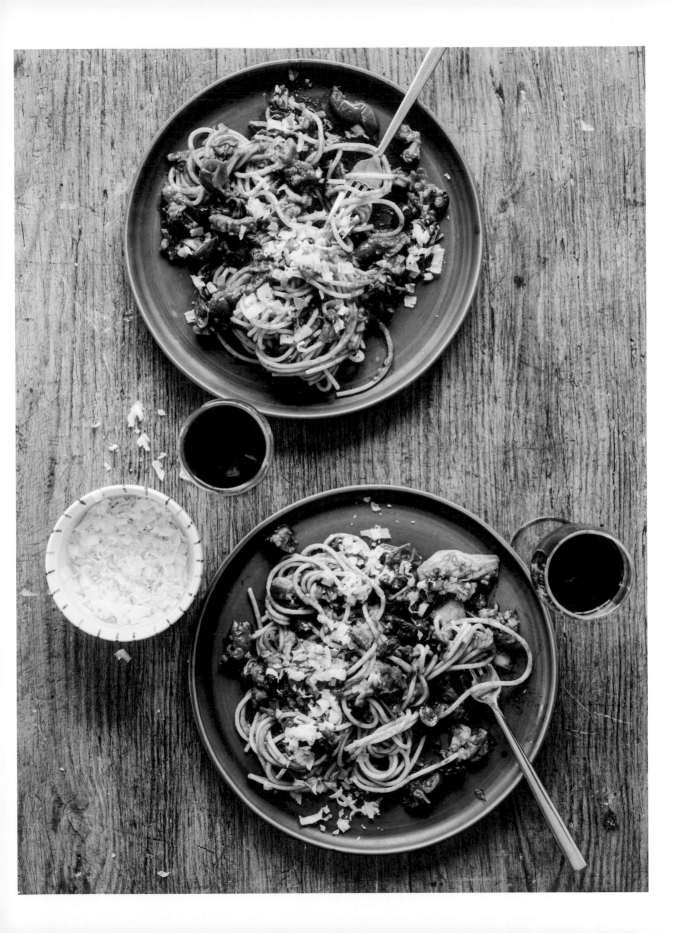

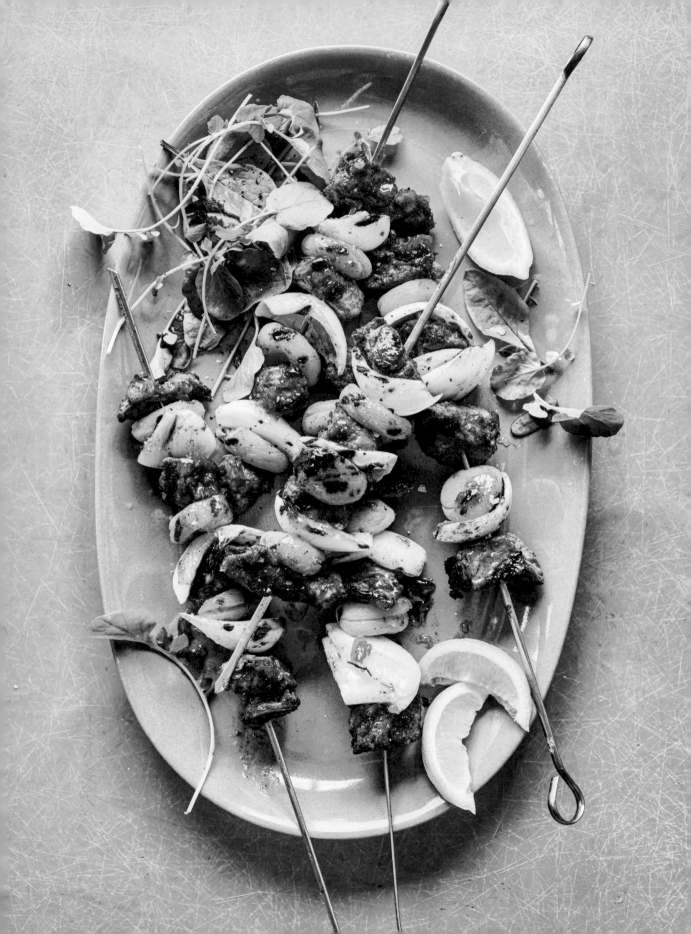

FRUITY-TOOTY LAMB SKEWERS

Serves 4
302 calories

We were going to call these tutti-frutti skewers but had visions of everyone looking crestfallen when they realized we weren't talking of either ice cream or those awful sweets your nana would buy you instead of wine gums. Just me? These skewers are great for throwing on the edge of a BBQ, though they'll cook just as well under the grill.

You mustn't limit this recipe to our suggestions either – you can throw pretty much any old tut on a skewer and make yourself a meal. If I may offer three tips: invest in metal skewers (or soak some wooden ones) before you start (and then subsequently forget how bloody hot they get as they melt through your hand). Also, chop all your vegetables to roughly the same size before skewering. It's common sense, but you'd be amazed how many times Paul gets it wrong. Feel free to substitute the lamb for pork or chicken or, if you're wanting to go entirely meat-free, whack on the old faithful: halloumi with a squeeze of lemon.

1 onion, quartered, plus ¼ onion, finely diced
1 clove of garlic, finely chopped
1 teaspoon grated ginger
2 tablespoons sugar-free apricot jam
2 tablespoons cider vinegar
1 tablespoon curry powder
½ tablespoon garam masala
450g (1lb) lamb, cut into 2cm (¾ inch) cubes
16 dried apricots

Heat a small pan over a medium heat and spray with a little oil. Add the finely diced onion and cook until softened. Add the garlic and ginger and cook for a minute, then add the jam, vinegar, curry powder and garam masala and stir well. Remove from the heat and set aside until cooled.

Tip the lamb into a bowl and pour over the marinade. Mix well, then cover and leave in the fridge for a few hours, or overnight if you can.

When you're ready to assemble the skewers, pour hot (but not boiling) water over the apricots until covered and allow them to soften for about 15 minutes, then drain.

Divide the onion quarters into separate layers. Remove the cubes of lamb from the fridge and thread them on to skewers, alternating with pieces of onion and plumped-up apricots, repeating until everything is used up.

Place under a high grill or on a barbecue for about 15–20 minutes, until the lamb is cooked through.

Notes from Paul
- Sugar-free jam will keep the calories low – but normal jam will work fine too.
- Reduce the curry powder if you don't like it too spicy – or increase it if you want it spicier!

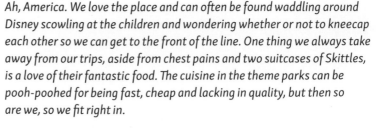

A PAN FULL OF SLOPPY JOE

Serves 6
488 calories

Ah, America. We love the place and can often be found waddling around Disney scowling at the children and wondering whether or not to kneecap each other so we can get to the front of the line. One thing we always take away from our trips, aside from chest pains and two suitcases of Skittles, is a love of their fantastic food. The cuisine in the theme parks can be pooh-poohed for being fast, cheap and lacking in quality, but then so are we, so we fit right in.

A sloppy joe is delicious – a sandwich stuffed full of seasoned beef mince. A hamburger that will leave your shirt stained, your beard wet and your belly full. We've combined it with potatoes and cooked it all in one pan to try to minimize the fuss, and the resulting dish is absolutely glorious!

900g (2lb) potatoes, cut into 1cm (½ inch) cubes
1 tablespoon olive oil
2 teaspoons Worcestershire sauce
1 onion, finely chopped
2 cloves of garlic, crushed
750g (1½lb) beef mince
500g (1lb 2oz/2 cups) passata
1 medium carrot, peeled and finely diced
1 red pepper, finely diced
2 celery stalks, finely diced
1 teaspoon mustard powder
1 teaspoon chilli powder
1 teaspoon cider vinegar
a good pinch of salt and freshly ground black pepper
80g (3oz/¾ cup) mozzarella cheese, grated
1 tablespoon hot sauce (we use Buffalo sauce, but feel free to mix it up)

Preheat the oven to 180°C fan/400°F/gas mark 6.

Pop the cubes of potato into a bowl with the olive oil and Worcestershire sauce and tumble them around until nicely coated. Scatter them on a baking sheet and cook in the oven for 35–45 minutes, turning them every now and then until they've softened and browned.

While the potatoes are cooking, heat a little oil in a pan over a medium heat and cook your onion, adding the garlic just as the onion is turning translucent.

Add the beef mince and cook until browned.

Add the passata, carrot, red pepper and celery and stir through, then stir in the mustard powder, chilli powder, cider vinegar, salt, pepper and a tablespoon of water. Cover the pan and allow to bubble away gently on a medium heat until everything has thickened up nicely.

When the potatoes are ready, stir them straight into the pan and make sure everything is mixed together well.

Top with the mozzarella, or any other cheese you've got to hand, and pop under the grill until the cheese has browned nicely.

Drizzle with the hot sauce and serve.

Notes from Paul
- *If you have an air fryer, pop the potato cubes in with a dash of oil and the Worcestershire sauce – the air fryer will take care of them, tumbling as necessary.*
- *If you use a large, ovenproof frying pan, this whole dish becomes a one-pot job.*
- *If you're not planning on having your 'I'm being good' side salad with this, it will make enough for four big portions.*

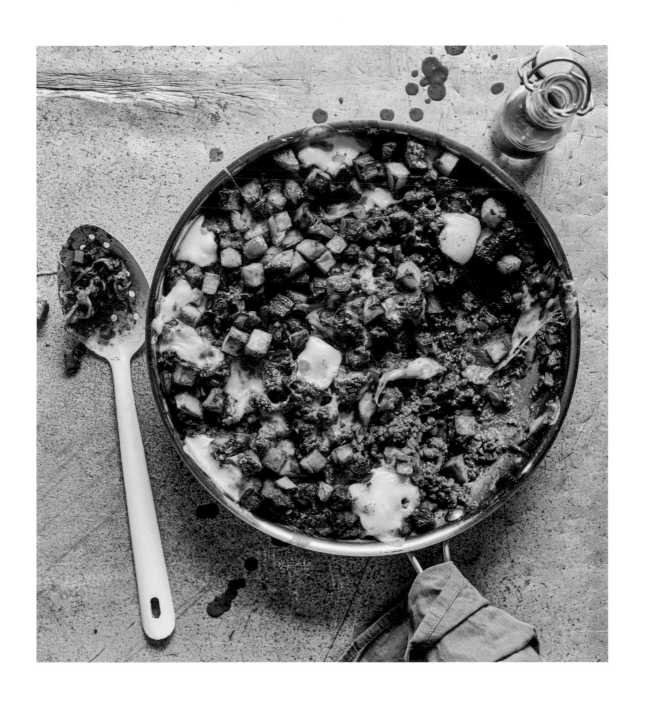

NO NEED TO PEEL THE POTATOES, BUT YOU CAN IF YOU PREFER — WE'RE ALL ABOUT THE RUSTIC LOOK HERE AT TWOCHUBBYCUBS, WHICH GOES SOME WAY TO EXPLAINING PAUL'S FACE.

GROATY PUDDING (A SLOW-COOKED ONE-POT WONDER!)

Serves 4
493 calories

Throughout this book we have popped in recipes from our travels, and it would seem remiss not to include Birmingham in those international travels of ours. Birmingham, though? See, we ended up in Birmingham entirely by accident on day one of our pledge to lose all the weight. We had (unadvisedly) booked ourselves on to a coach trip which turned into quite the endurance feat, and, in a fit of temper at being asked to eat our dinner from a trestle table in a budget hotel, we ditched the whole affair and made our own arrangements to get back.

The best part of this tale is the fact that we ended up at Cadbury World, where we had to record our first piece to camera with faces full of solemnity and determination about our weight loss. That's tricky to do when your pockets are sagging with the weight of four Double Deckers.

Now, in the spirit of finding a recipe from the Black Country to celebrate, we happened across this dish: a perfect marriage of lazy cooking (five minutes to prepare) and slovenly housekeeping (all cooked in one pot). We serve this over mustardy mashed potato and it really is just the thing for curling up with.

The traditional recipe calls for groats, but we'll be buggered if we can find them anywhere outside of health shops we're too intimidated to go into. We're reassured that pearl barley or even bog-standard oats will cut the mustard just as easy. We've tinkered with the recipe because we're cads and each love to get more vegetables in when the other isn't looking.

500g (1lb 2oz) or so of beef shin, chopped into chunks
2 white onions, chopped
3 leeks, chopped
1 of those bags of pre-chopped swede and carrot
250g (9oz/1¼ cups) pearl barley
600ml (20fl oz/2½ cups) beef stock
1 teaspoon Marmite

Prepare yourself for this one, mind, it's a complex affair.

Tip all your ingredients into a decent non-stick casserole dish, give everything a good stir, cover and place in the bottom of your oven on 160°C fan/350°F/gas mark 4 for a good 8 hours.

Do check on this dish regularly to make sure it hasn't boiled dry – you're looking for a thick, sticky, stodgy stew.

Serve, to the unending praise of your loved ones.

Notes from Paul
- *If you're not a fan of Marmite – and mind, that's enough cause for a wrestle in our house – leave it out and swap in a tablespoon or two of Worcestershire sauce.*
- *You could add a wee glass of Guinness if you were feeling decadent.*
- *If you can't get beef shin, panic not – use stewing steak, though don't necessarily go for the leanest because the fat helps with the flavour.*
- *Absolutely chuck this in a slow cooker if you like – it'll take a bit longer, and watch it doesn't catch.*

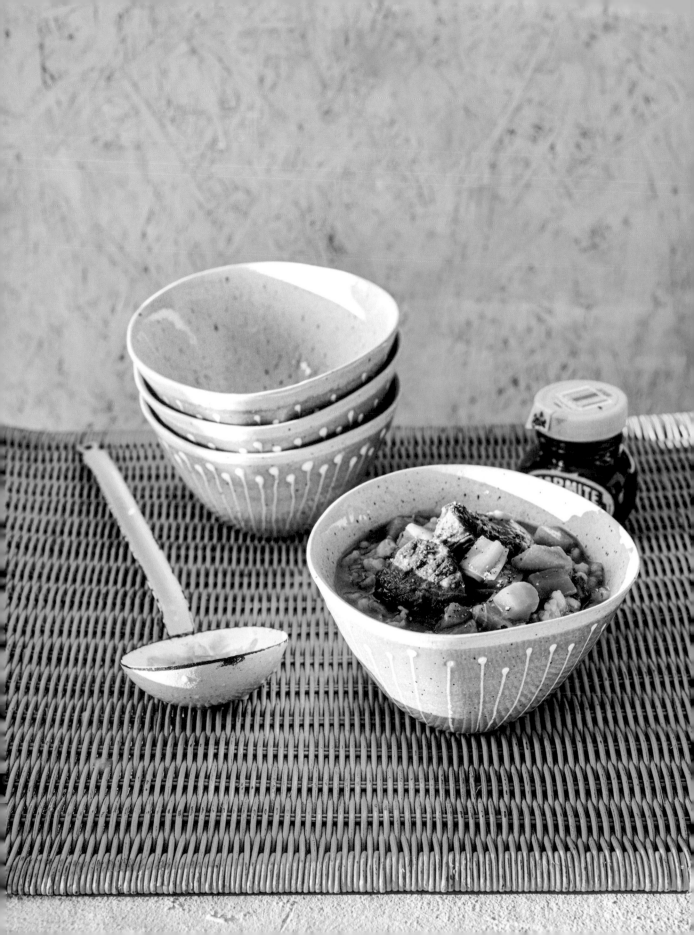

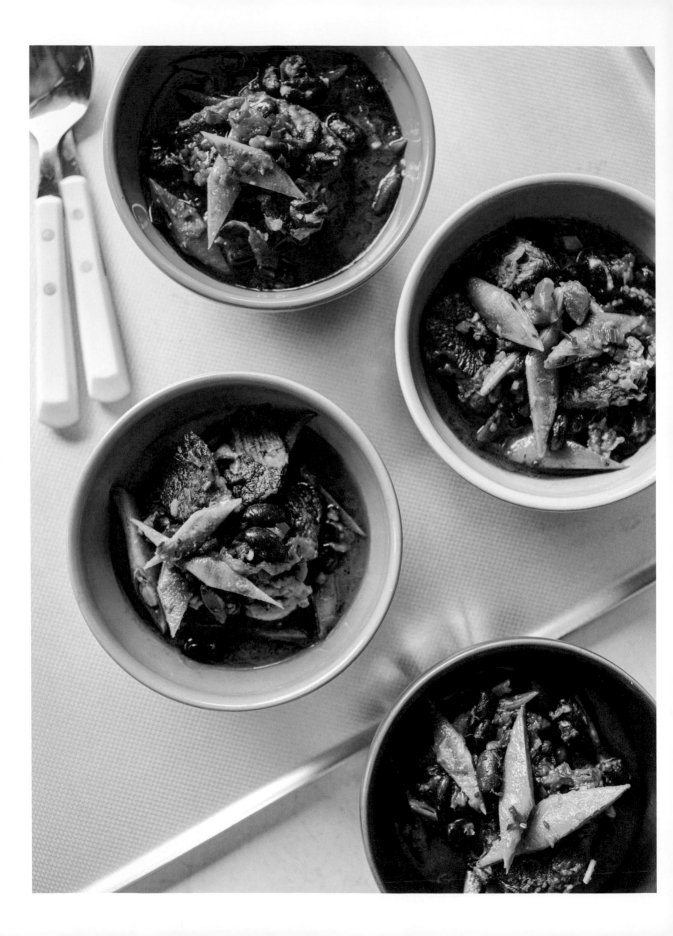

SPICY MEXICAN BEEF

Serves 4
499 calories

1kg (2lb 3oz) stewing beef, cut
     into large chunks
2 onions, chopped
6 cloves of garlic, finely chopped
450g (1lb) tomatoes, deseeded
     and chopped
2 red chillies, deseeded and
     thinly sliced
1 tablespoon chipotle paste
1.5 litres (2¾ pints/6 cups)
     beef stock
1 × 400g (14oz) tin of red kidney
     beans, drained and rinsed
325g (12½oz) frozen runner
     beans

Spicy Mexican Beef – this is a cheery dish that you can cobble together in one pan and just leave to burble and simmer for an hour or two while you sit and cut your toenails.

If you're having a bad day because the world is getting on your boobs, we hear you. That's why a dish like this is for you: minimal effort, but still tastes bloody good. Serve with some rice – hell, with the mood you're in, we won't challenge you if you want to use microwave rice.

Heat a frying pan over a high heat and spray with a little oil. Add the beef to the pan and brown on all sides.

Reduce the heat to medium, add the onions and garlic, and stir constantly for 2 minutes.

Add the tomatoes, chillies, chipotle paste, beef stock and red kidney beans, then cover and simmer over a low heat for 1 hour and 15 minutes.

Add the runner beans, cook for a further 15 minutes, then serve.

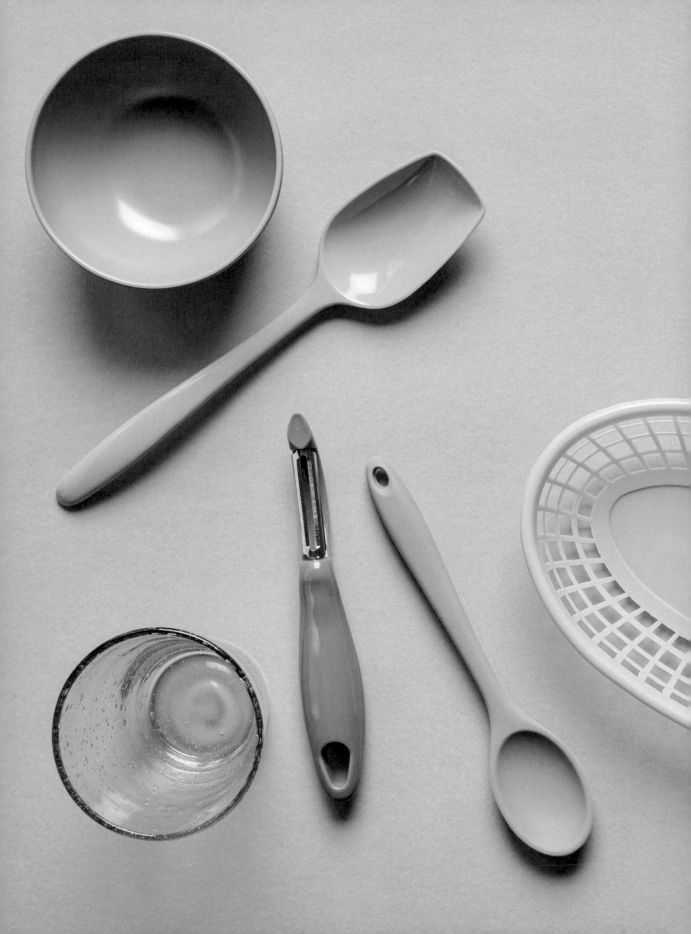

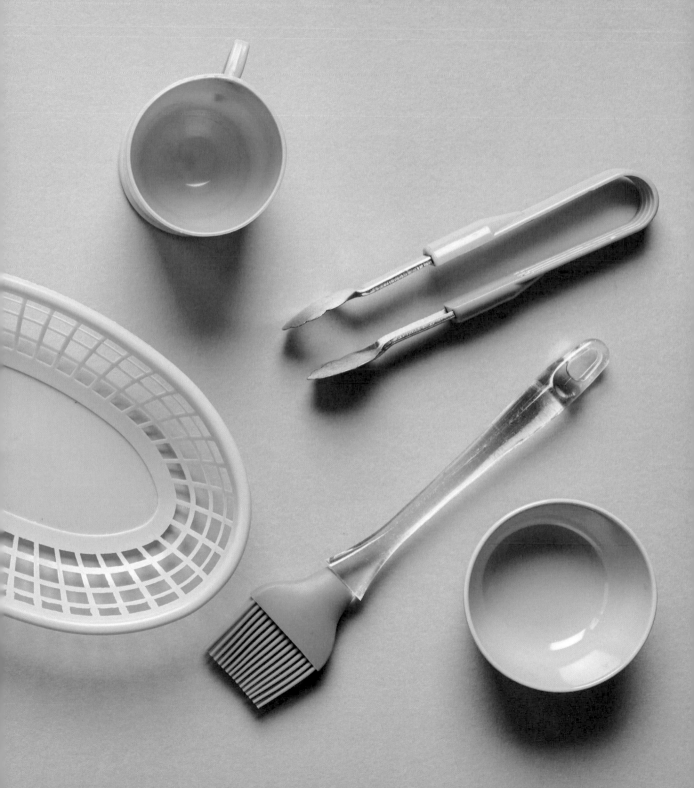

FAKEAWAYS

● ● ● ● ● ●

FISH CURRY

Serves 4
178 calories

The running theme through this book is that we aren't keen on fish; however, we're also endless adventurers and by that token, will give anything a go once. Firm believers in the fact you can't say you don't enjoy something until you've tried it, at least when it comes to food. So, to that end, if you're out there and going 'urgh' at the thought of this simple, light fish curry, I implore you to at least try it. Choose good fresh fish if you can.

I'd offer to pick you some up, but I'm absolutely not made for the sea. I can't handle ferry travel – I spend most of my time listing away on the deck trying not to vomit. I get dizzy reaching behind me for the toilet roll – don't add a rolling ocean into that. Even below the surface I'm no better. We tried 'scuba diving' a few years ago – all was well until I realized I was following someone who clearly forgot herself and merrily took a slash as she sauntered along underwater. I made anemone for life there.

Oh! And side note: if you're large and wet-suit clad, fair warning: when it comes to taking the bloody thing off, you'll be there for a good twenty minutes, nineteen of which will be spent trying to stifle your giggles at the giant sucky fart noises that come from peeling it off afterwards.

Fish curry then …

1 onion, finely chopped
4 cloves of garlic, crushed
2.5cm (1 inch) ginger, peeled and grated
2 teaspoons ground coriander
1 teaspoon ground cumin
½ teaspoon paprika
½ teaspoon ground turmeric
½ teaspoon mustard seeds
½ teaspoon cayenne pepper
2 tomatoes, finely diced
250ml (9fl oz/1 cup) light coconut milk
2 green chillies, sliced
450g (1lb) white fish, cut into 2cm (¾ inch) pieces
1 tablespoon lime juice

Heat a large saucepan over a medium heat and spray it with some oil. Add the onion and fry gently until turning golden, then reduce the heat to medium and add the garlic, ginger, coriander, cumin, paprika, turmeric, mustard seeds and cayenne pepper. Stir continuously for 1 minute.

Add the tomatoes and cook for 3–4 minutes, then pour in the coconut milk. Add the sliced chillies and 120ml (4fl oz/½ cup) of water and bring to the boil, then reduce to a simmer. Cover the pan and cook for 10–15 minutes.

Add the fish and cook for about 6–8 minutes, until firm.

Add the lime juice, stir well and serve.

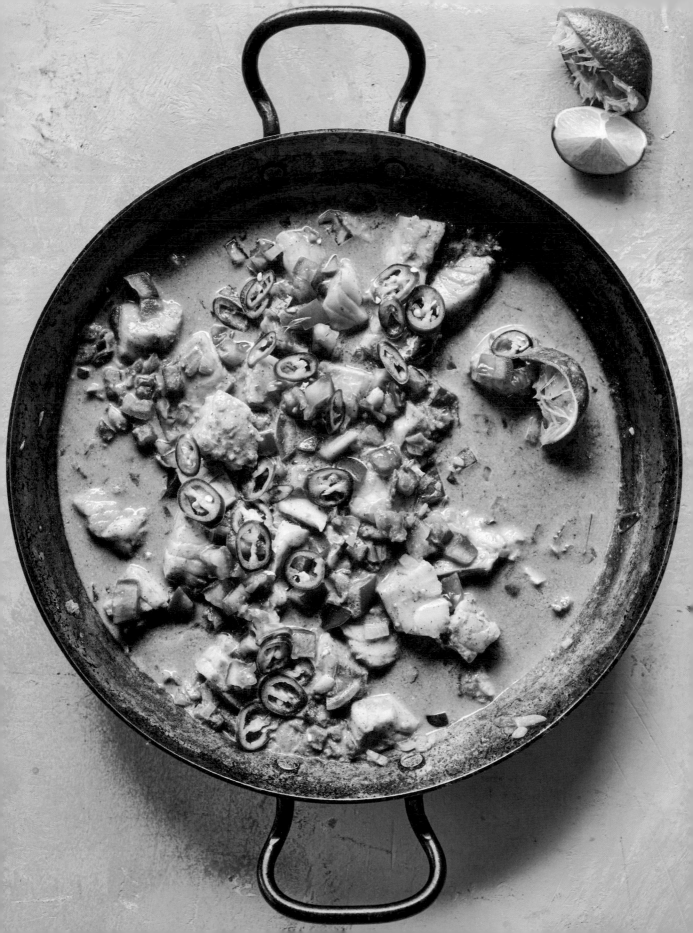

● ● ● ● ●

TANDOORI CHICKEN BURGER

Serves 4
498 calories

We wrestled with our conscience about putting this in the book: neither of us are particular fans of 'burgers' that aren't burgers at all. You know the sort: a brioche bun (sorry, are we having breakfast?), a slab of gristle and then a whole weekly food-shop of toppings. You know you're into mischief territory when it comes on a wooden board with a spike down the middle, holding everything together.

I mean, what's the point? I'm not a bloody anaconda. Heston Blumenthal – a man who actually bewitches me when he talks – has a three-finger rule: anything taller than the height of three of your fingers pressed together will cause your jaw to ache. He's absolutely bang on, and so, when it comes to assembling this burger, don't go doolally with the toppings. Leave them wanting more! And if you're struggling with the bhajis, fret not – press them into a muffin tray. They'll cook just fine.

4 skinless, boneless chicken
  breasts
4 tablespoons fat-free yoghurt
2 teaspoons mint sauce
4 × 57g (2oz) burger buns
4 tablespoons mango chutney
½ a cucumber, sliced

For the tandoori marinade
1 tablespoon ground coriander
1 tablespoon ground cumin
2 teaspoons hot chilli powder
1 teaspoon ground turmeric
1 teaspoon mint sauce
2 teaspoons curry powder
2 teaspoons ground fenugreek
2 tablespoons tandoori paste
4 cloves of garlic, crushed
2.5cm (1 inch) ginger, peeled and
  very finely chopped

For the onion bhajis
3 brown onions, thinly sliced
3 tablespoons chickpea flour
2 teaspoons tomato purée
½ teaspoon ground cumin
½ teaspoon ground coriander

Put all the marinade ingredients into a bowl along with 75ml (2½fl oz/ ⅓ cup) of water and mix really well. Pop the chicken breasts into the bowl and mix well so all the chicken breasts are covered. Cover with cling film and leave to marinate in the fridge for at least an hour, or ideally overnight.

Preheat the oven to 200°C fan/425°F/gas mark 7 and line a baking sheet with greaseproof paper.

To make the bhajis, heat a large frying pan over a medium heat and spray with a little oil. Add the onions and stir well, then keep stirring occasionally until they start to soften and go translucent. Remove from the heat, add the rest of the bhaji ingredients to the pan along with 1 tablespoon of water, and stir well.

Spoon the onion mixture onto the lined baking sheet, using 2 tablespoons per dollop, and flatten each dollop into a small burger shape. Spray with a bit of oil and bake in the oven for 45 minutes.

While the bhajis are baking, preheat the grill to medium-high and cook the chicken breasts until done.

Mix together the yoghurt and mint sauce, and slice the buns in half horizontally. Spread the mango chutney evenly over each bottom half, then spoon some of the yoghurt sauce on top. Place the cucumber on top of the yoghurt. Top each one with a cooked chicken breast and an onion bhaji. Finish with some more sauce, if desired, and the top halves of the buns.

Note from Paul
Don't be scared of the flour in the bhajis – it'll help give that proper bhaji mouthfeel and taste.

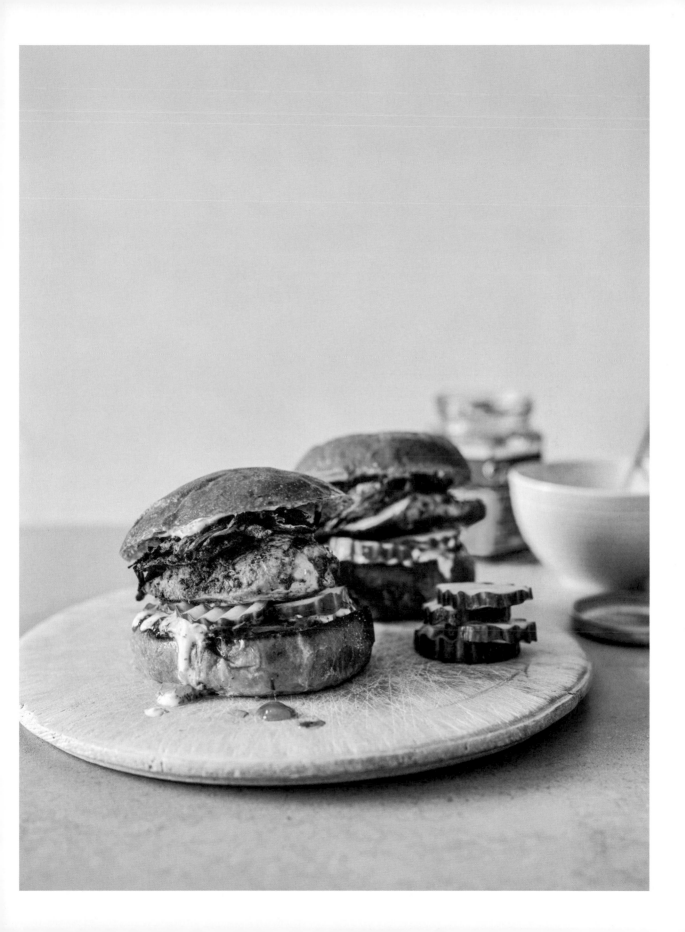

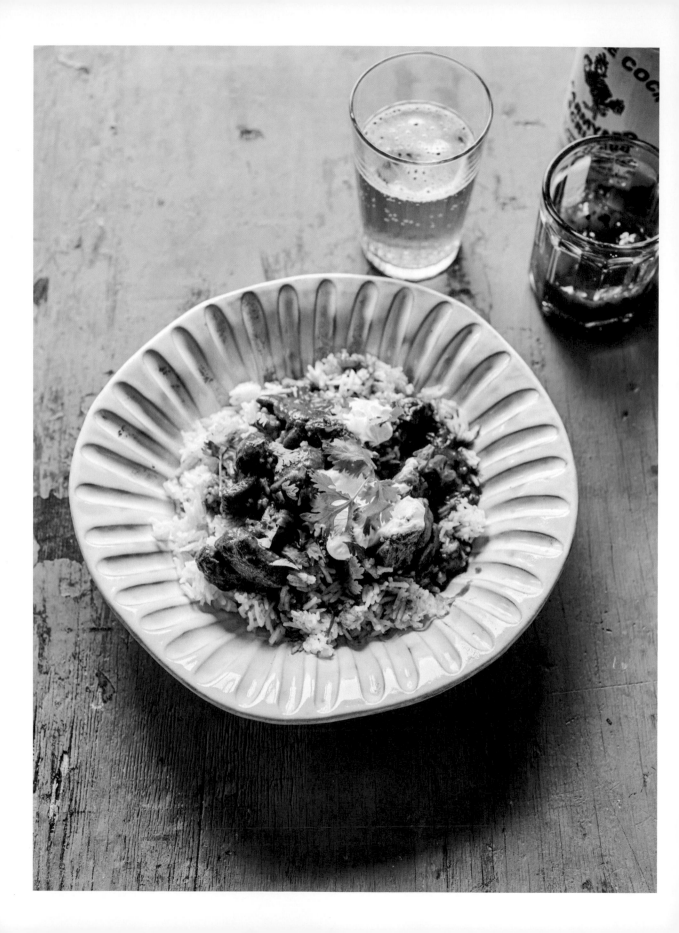

CHICKEN TIKKA MASALA

• • • • • •

Serves 4
457 calories

Sometimes you need a faithful recipe to come home to of an evening, and this is very much one of those: a reliable chuck-what-you-like-in curry that you can make with bits you'll have at home. I'm going to open the recipe with a plea: don't swap out the coconut milk for a coconut-scented yoghurt. I shouldn't have to say this, no, but by gum I do – years of experience in the slimming groups has taught me that if someone can ruin a recipe in the pursuit of a 'free' dinner, they bloody well will.

We're not about that at Twochubbycubs, no: what's better for you? A meal you enjoy because it tastes like it should and just happens to be healthy, or a meal you've cobbled together from hotchpotch ingredients that taste disgusting but you can kid yourself it's tasty because 'no fats'? Hmm? If your answer is the latter rather than the former then I shall politely ask you to close this book and never return.

No, no such tut with Twochubbycubs, so please take heed: use the coconut milk. Or so help me …

750g (1½lb) skinless, boneless chicken thighs, diced
1 teaspoon ground turmeric
2 teaspoons ground cumin
2 teaspoons garam masala
1 teaspoon ground coriander
½ teaspoon black pepper
¼ teaspoon cayenne pepper
1 teaspoon paprika
2 tablespoons olive oil
1 onion, chopped
4 cloves of garlic, crushed
2.5cm (1 inch) ginger, peeled and grated
4 tablespoons tomato purée
200g (7oz) tinned chopped tomatoes
1 × 400ml (14fl oz) tin of light coconut milk
250ml (9fl oz/1 cup) chicken stock
½ teaspoon crushed chilli flakes

Put the chicken into a bowl. Mix together the turmeric, ground cumin, garam masala, ground coriander, black pepper, cayenne pepper and paprika and sprinkle over the chicken. Mix well, ensuring that the chicken is well coated.

Heat a large frying pan over a medium-high heat and add the olive oil. Add the chicken and cook until no pink meat remains, then remove from the pan and set aside.

Add the chopped onion to the same pan and stir until golden brown. Add the garlic and ginger and cook for a minute or 2, then add the tomato purée and stir well. Add the chopped tomatoes and stir again, then stir in the coconut milk, followed by the chicken stock. Simmer over a medium-low heat for 14 minutes.

Dice the chicken and add to the pan along with the chilli flakes. Simmer for another 10–15 minutes, then serve.

Note from Paul
We use chicken thighs because they give a richer taste and texture, but chicken breasts would work just as well.

●●●●●●

CHUBBY BAKED CHICKEN

Serves 4
340 calories

We have been asked to replicate the chicken of a certain fast-food retailer many times over, and, well, we like a challenge. This is the closest we have ever managed to come to getting the ingredients just right, although I'm sure the Colonel might have something to say about it.

Now, you might despair at the long list of herbs and spices and rightly so – if this is the first time you're having to schlep out and buy them, it's a big commitment. But here's the thing: if you're cooking your own meals, they're all ingredients that you will use over and over. Well, maybe not marjoram, we're still not convinced that's not just someone having a joke, but still … Keep your spices in a good airtight tin and they'll last, but not for ever: don't be afraid to chuck them out once they've lost their pungency and colour.

We had a moment in IKEA a few months ago and ended up buying fifty tiny airproof tins that stick to the side of the fridge to keep our spices in. It looks great, although the fact we have a tin full of sprinkles and another tin full of hundreds and thousands perhaps tells you exactly how seriously we take our dieting.

100g (3½oz/1½ cups) panko
    breadcrumbs
3 eggs
5 chicken thighs or 4 chicken
    breasts, skinless and boneless

For the spices
2 tablespoons onion granules
1 tablespoon salt
1 tablespoon black pepper
1 tablespoon garlic granules
1 tablespoon dried thyme
1 tablespoon dried sage
1 tablespoon dried marjoram
1 tablespoon dried mixed herbs
1 tablespoon ground ginger
1 tablespoon paprika
1 tablespoon mustard powder
1 tablespoon cayenne pepper

Preheat the oven to 200°C fan/425°F/gas mark 7 and spray a baking sheet with a few sprays of oil.

Mix the panko and all the spices together in a bowl – don't be afraid to grind the breadcrumbs a little to make sure everything is combined.

Crack the eggs into a bowl and beat well.

Dip the chicken in the egg and allow any excess to drip off, then roll the egg-covered chicken in the panko and spice mix until well coated – feel free to use your fingers to pack extra coating into every nook and cranny.

Pop the coated chicken pieces onto the baking sheet and put them into the oven for 35–40 minutes, until cooked through.

Notes from Paul
- *If you have an air fryer, take the paddle out and cook them in there.*
- *You could use chicken strips for this and make chicken fingers, which we are reassured are real things.*
- *The spice mix can be kept in an airtight jar (though obviously not after you've dipped your egg in it).*
- *Can't be chewed on buying all of the herbs and spices? That's fine, just find a Cajun spice mix in the supermarket.*

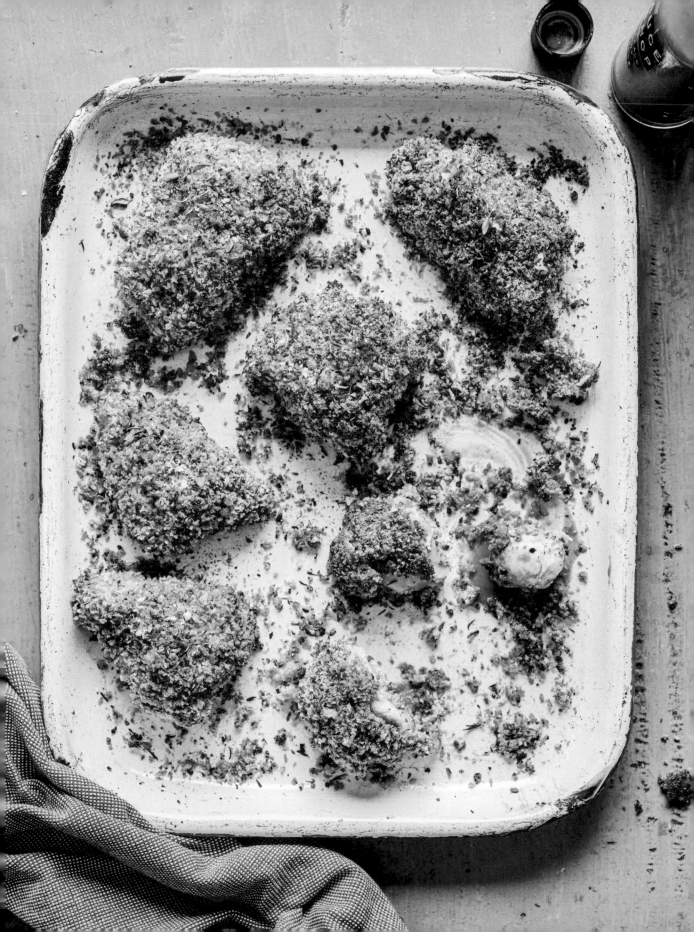

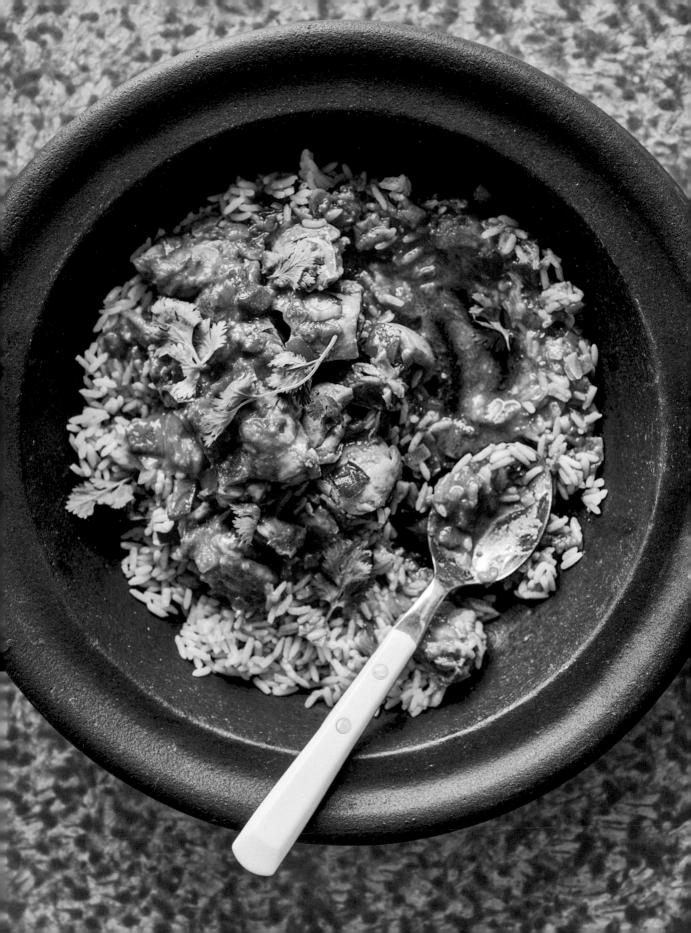

QUICK & EASY CHICKEN CURRY

Serves 4
288 calories

We confess to not being especially adventurous when it comes to curries – there's always that angst about ordering something that comes burning a hole through the plate and then having to eat it because a) you've paid for it and b) the restaurant owner is gazing at you with wounded eyes in case you don't like his food. Seriously: we have a fabulous Indian restaurant near us where the owner does exactly that – sits at the top table watching everyone eat. It's become a test of endurance that I could do without, if I'm frank, but Paul is ever hopeful that he's going to get noticed.

To that end, I'm equally as hopeful.

We hope you'll forgive us this simple recipe, but we've learnt over time that if we create a fabulously exciting recipe with all sorts of spices, people tend to tune out. So actually, you only have yourselves to blame. As this is low in calories and high in taste, we tend to serve it with simple boiled rice and plenty of scoopy breads on the side. 'Tis yours to do with as you wish.

2 large white onions, finely chopped
1 large red pepper, finely chopped
2 tablespoons garlic and ginger paste
5 skinless, boneless chicken thighs, diced into small chunks
1 × 400g (14oz) tin of chopped tomatoes
1 × 400ml (14fl oz) tin of light coconut milk
1 tablespoon curry powder
200ml (7fl oz/¾ cup) chicken stock
1 tablespoon tomato purée

Cook the onions and pepper low and slow in a non-stick frying pan until golden, adding the ginger and garlic paste towards the end.

Push the onions and pepper to one side of the pan and throw in the chicken, cooking until it's sealed.

Add everything else to the pan and leave to bubble and simmer for about 25 minutes, until the sauce has reduced and is delicious and thick.

Notes from Paul
- *Lots of folk swap out coconut milk for coconut yoghurt – for the love of everything dear to you, don't do it. Using the proper ingredients makes it taste so much better.*
- *The longer you leave everything to gently bubble, the thicker and sweeter the sauce will be.*

• • • • • •

ONE POT PHO

Serves 4
393 calories

1 onion, cut into quarters
5cm (2 inches) ginger, peeled and
    sliced thinly
3 cloves of garlic, crushed
3 cloves
2 star anise
1 cinnamon stick
1 teaspoon ground coriander
10 cardamom pods
1 teaspoon black peppercorns
6 skinless, boneless chicken
    thighs
2 chicken stock cubes
2 tablespoons fish sauce
1 teaspoon brown sugar
240g (8½oz) rice noodles
100g (3½oz/1 cup) ready-to-eat
    beansprouts

To serve
10 fresh basil leaves
10 fresh mint leaves, sliced
1 red chilli, thinly sliced
1 lime, cut into wedges

I bloody love pho: it's one of those dishes I'll always try to order if I find it on a menu. Well, not strictly true, it's certainly one of those dishes I'll want to order but end up agonizing over how to pronounce it before I crumble and order something I can say without the waiter snickering into his sleeve. It's pronounced 'fuh' apparently, though I'll forget that by the end of this sentence …

You don't need a pressure cooker for this, you can do just as well on the hob. A pressure cooker makes light work of it, however, so if you're on the fence, this might tempt you over. There's a load of pressure cooker ideas on the blog if you're stuck. As with all of our recipes, feel free to add whatever you like into this – it's a soup after all, it can take it.

Set a pressure cooker to the sauté setting and spray with a little oil. Add the onion, ginger and garlic and stir continuously for 3–4 minutes.

Add the cloves, star anise, cinnamon stick, ground coriander, cardamom pods and peppercorns and cook for another minute.

Turn off the pressure cooker, then add the chicken thighs, crumbled stock cubes, fish sauce and sugar. Pour in 1.5 litres (2¾ pints/6 cups) of boiling water and give everything a good stir. Select the manual setting on the pressure cooker and cook for 15 minutes under high pressure.

When finished, use the quick-release. Remove the chicken from the pan, pull apart with 2 forks and set aside. Pour the liquid through a sieve and chuck out any solids that are left. Put the pulled chicken back into the soup.

Cook the noodles in a large pan of boiling water according to the packet instructions, then drain.

Add the noodles to the soup along with the beansprouts and ladle into bowls. Top with the basil leaves and the sliced mint and chillies, and serve with a lime wedge on the side.

Note from Paul
Chicken breasts will work just as well in this, or even some thinly sliced pork, if you have some.

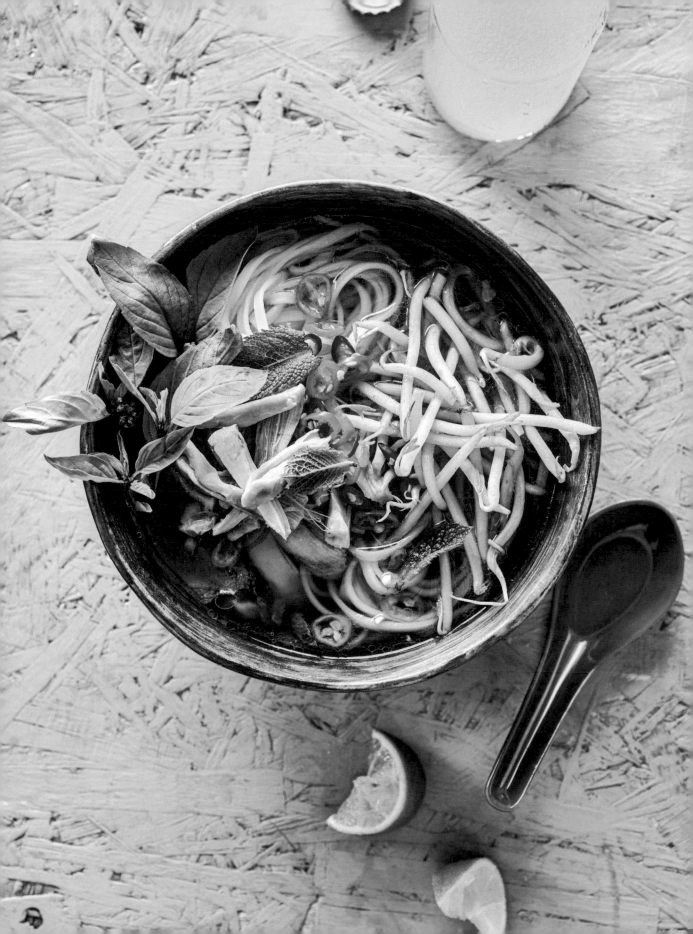

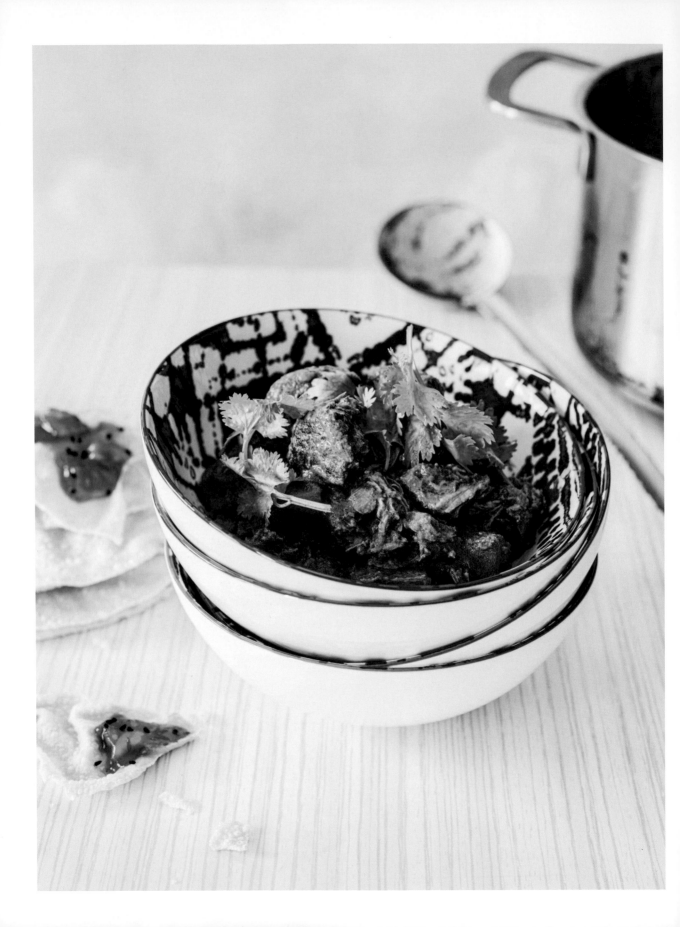

PROPER LAMB ROGAN JOSH

Serves 4
499 calories

1 red onion, finely diced
½ teaspoon cayenne pepper
1 teaspoon paprika
1½ teaspoon garam masala
4 cloves of garlic
2.5cm (1 inch) ginger, peeled and grated
1 teaspoon ground coriander
¼ teaspoon ground turmeric
800g (1lb 12oz) diced lamb
125g (4½oz/½ cup) yoghurt (see note)
2 potatoes, cut into 2cm (¾ inch) cubes

As mentioned earlier in the book, we love Birmingham. The last time we were down we went for an amazing curry with two good friends, who we then returned the favour to by showing them around Newcastle. They loved it – but who wouldn't, with Paul and I showing you around while making catty asides to each other?

Newcastle is a terrific city full of genuine pleasures. We have good food – from the saveloy dip to Michelin-starred restaurants. Well, one at the time of writing. But it counts! The nightlife is superb, so I'm told – I'm too old for anything other than a milk stout and a couple of hands of Solitaire. And the people, oh the people: friendly without being fake, fun without being jolly-hockey about it. It's a welcoming little secret and I heartily encourage anyone to visit and see for themselves. I love to travel, but I adore coming huurm (home).

Anyway, that's enough from me on Newcastle. With the recipe, please do go for full-fat yoghurt. The recipe tastes all the better for it.

Heat a large frying pan over a medium heat, then spray it with a little oil and add the onion. Fry until golden brown, which will take about 8–10 minutes.

In a small bowl mix the cayenne pepper and paprika with 2 tablespoons of water, to make a paste. Add the paste to the frying pan along with the garam masala, garlic, ginger, coriander and turmeric, and stir well for 1 minute.

Add the diced lamb to the pan and cook over a medium heat until hardly any pink remains. Reduce the heat to low and cook for a few more minutes, until the lamb is no longer pink and the outside of the meat is slightly browned.

Add the yoghurt to the pan, a couple of tablespoons at a time, and stir well. Remove the pan from the heat.

Transfer everything to a slow cooker and add the potatoes, along with 250ml (9fl oz/1 cup) of water. Cover and cook on low for 5 hours.

If you don't have a slow cooker, you can cook this in a lidded casserole dish in the oven at 180°C fan/400°F/gas mark 6 for 30 minutes. Don't add the yoghurt until just before serving. Serve with rice.

Note from Paul
Don't use fat-free yoghurt in this because it will curdle. Spring for the standard version instead because it will taste nicer and cook better. You aren't using a huge amount so don't worry too much about the calories – it will be worth it.

● ● ● ● ● ●

MONGOLIAN BEEF

Serves 4
287 calories

500g (1lb 2oz) beef steak, sliced
as thinly as you dare –
or, to save a bit of time,
buy beef strips
25g (1oz/3 tablespoons) cornflour
a few good twists of black pepper
3 cloves of garlic, crushed
½ teaspoon finely grated ginger
120ml (4fl oz/½ cup) low-sodium
soy sauce
25g (1oz/2½ tablespoons) brown
sugar
1 teaspoon chilli flakes
3 spring onions, finely sliced

One little faux-pas that we made on the blog back in the early days was not realizing that the images we use in the accompanying story carry through on to social media whenever you post a link to a recipe. That's usually fine – who doesn't like looking at my buttocks while they try to find a recipe for carrot dip – but not for this one. We had prattled on about volunteering at our local cat and dog shelter and included a picture of a lovely wee Jack Russell. Problem is, whenever we post this recipe for 'quick takeaway beef', a picture of a sad-looking dog pops up, leading to us having to feverishly explain that we're not chopping up Rex for a 'fakeaway' recipe.

This recipe gets pulled out over and over by our followers and we know exactly why – it's a fakeaway recipe that takes no time to make, doesn't have a huge list of ingredients and tastes amazing. You might be tempted to swap the sugar for sweetener but you mustn't – it'll taste like crap. Remember: food is there to be enjoyed, not endured!

Place the beef on some kitchen paper and dry it off. Pop it into a bowl with the cornflour and pepper and toss until it is evenly covered, then set aside.

In a good non-stick pan, heat a little oil over a medium heat and gently cook the garlic and ginger until coloured, but be careful not to burn them. Add the soy sauce, brown sugar, chilli flakes and 120ml (4fl oz/ ½ cup) of water and cook until everything has thickened down nicely.

Pour the sauce into a jug. Put the beef straight into the same pan and cook on high until browned on all sides.

Pour the sauce over the beef and allow to bubble for a minute or 2.

Sprinkle the spring onions over the top and serve with rice and a smile.

Note from Paul
We can't stress enough about using low-sodium soy sauce – swap it for normal sodium soy sauce and you'll have a mouth saltier than a sailor's ankle.

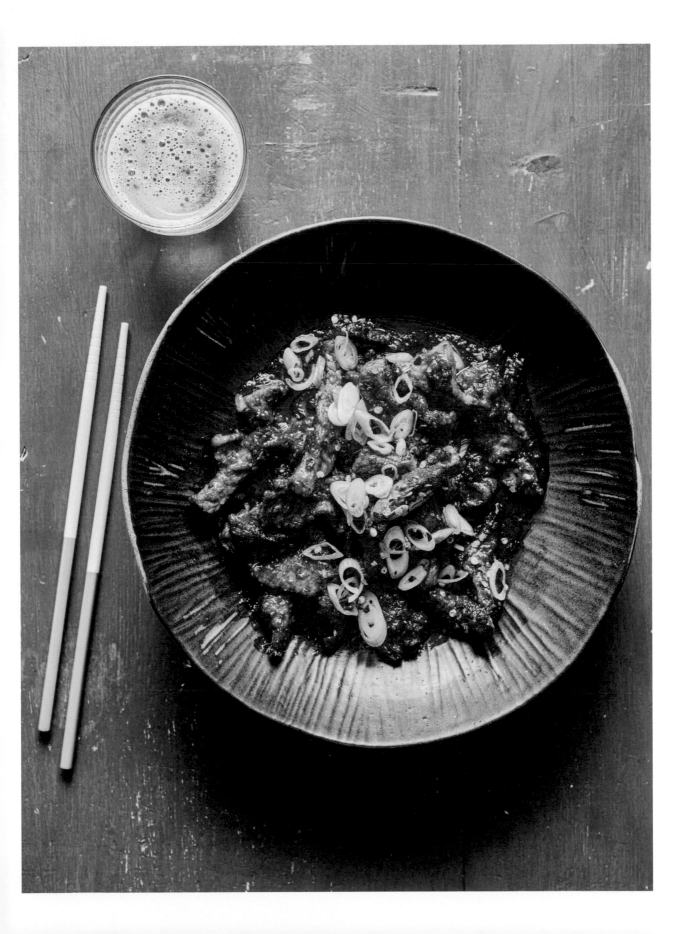

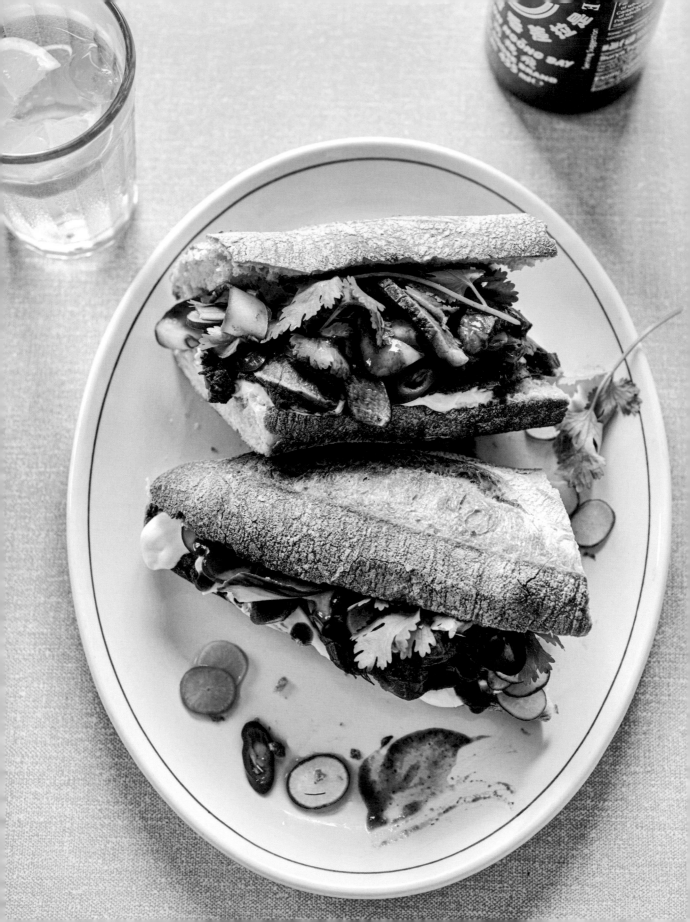

STEAK BANH MI

••••••

Serves 4
457 calories

Steak. It's an expensive ingredient, absolutely – but that's not to say you can't get away with using a slightly cheaper cut and cutting it fine. In fact, for this recipe at the very least, there's really no need to splash out on anything too expensive. It's a steak sandwich love, let's not get too excitable.

Paul is forever kvetching at me to save money but has lost the moral high-ground now he's discovered those websites that ship you all manner of tat from China for a couple of quid. He finds it difficult to tell me off for splashing the cash when envelopes full of light-up shoelaces, off-brand Simpsons memorabilia and 'REAL 100%' gold bars come tumbling through the door. We've had to pay off our postman as an apology for giving him a hernia.

You could do worse than brushing the bread with a little garlic oil and finishing it off under the grill before topping it. But, of course, you must watch those calories.

60ml (2fl oz/¼ cup) cider vinegar
2 tablespoons sugar
½ teaspoon coriander seeds
5 cardamom pods
2 teaspoons fresh dill leaves
8 radishes, thinly sliced
½ a cucumber, thinly sliced
2 part-baked baguettes
2 frying steaks
2 tablespoons reduced-fat mayonnaise
2 tablespoons fat-free natural yoghurt
2 red chillies, sliced
a handful of fresh coriander leaves
2 tablespoons sriracha
salt and freshly ground black pepper

Pour the vinegar and sugar into a pan along with the coriander seeds and cardamom pods and heat over a medium-low heat until the sugar has dissolved.

Add the dill, radishes and cucumber and cook for a few more minutes, then remove from the heat and set aside to cool.

Meanwhile, bake the baguettes according to the packet instructions and allow to cool, then slice in half to make 4.

Heat a frying pan over a medium heat with a little spray oil and fry the steaks to your liking. Remove from the pan and leave to rest for a few minutes, then slice.

Mix together the mayonnaise and yoghurt with a little salt and pepper. Slice each half baguette lengthways and spread with the mayonnaise mixture.

Top each sandwich with the beef, chillies, coriander leaves and the pickled veg, and drizzle over the sriracha.

Notes from Paul
- Baguettes work best for authenticity, but any kind of roll will be fine.
- Leave out the sriracha if you don't like it too spicy.

• • • • • •
SATAY BURGER

Serves 4
390 calories

We used to order a chicken satay almost weekly from our local Chinese takeaway – it was getting to the point where we'd ring up and, having seen our number pop up, they would answer the phone by confirming that our order was being prepared and would be ready to be picked up shortly. We were four more orders away from being invited to family weddings and having a plaque put above the door when disaster struck.

The council – in their infinite but shocking wisdom – decided that the takeaway deserved a one-star-out-of-five rating and frankly, this sent us into a tailspin of agonizing choice. Do you risk a week on the lavatory for the sake of a decent egg-fried rice? Does it <u>really</u> matter if the container walked to the bin of its own accord when you get two free bags of prawn crackers? Sadly, for Paul, it did matter, and the takeaway was binned off. We've never quite managed to get the fakeaway right but, with the need to scratch that peanut itch, we had to find an alternative.

And here it is! A beef satay burger – perhaps we're over-selling it, but the mix of savoury, salty and sweet is right up our street. It doesn't use a great deal of peanut butter either, so don't fret about getting your jeans buttoned up afterwards. It's worth every delicious bite!

4 tablespoons crunchy reduced-fat peanut butter
2 teaspoons light soy sauce
1 teaspoon dark soy sauce
2 tablespoons lime juice
500g (1lb 2oz) lean beef mince
4 baps
lettuce leaves
2 spring onions, sliced
2 red chillies, sliced

Mix together the peanut butter, soy sauces and lime juice in a bowl. Add a bit of water, a tablespoon at a time, until it reaches a ketchup-like consistency.

Tip the mince into a bowl and knead it a bit with your hands. Divide the mixture into 4, roll each piece into a ball and flatten down into a burger shape.

Heat a large frying pan over a high heat and spray with a little oil. Pop the burgers into the pan and cook for about 3–4 minutes on each side, or a little longer if you prefer them well done.

Slice the baps and place a few lettuce leaves on each of the bottom halves. Top with the burgers and spoon over the peanut sauce.

Sprinkle over the spring onions and chillies, add the tops of the baps, and serve.

Notes from Paul
- *You don't need to fanny on with adding breadcrumbs or cracking an egg into the mince to make burgers – it doesn't need it!*
- *Be careful not to over-knead the mince – just squeeze it a bit with your hands until it loses its 'strings' and stays in a big ball shape.*

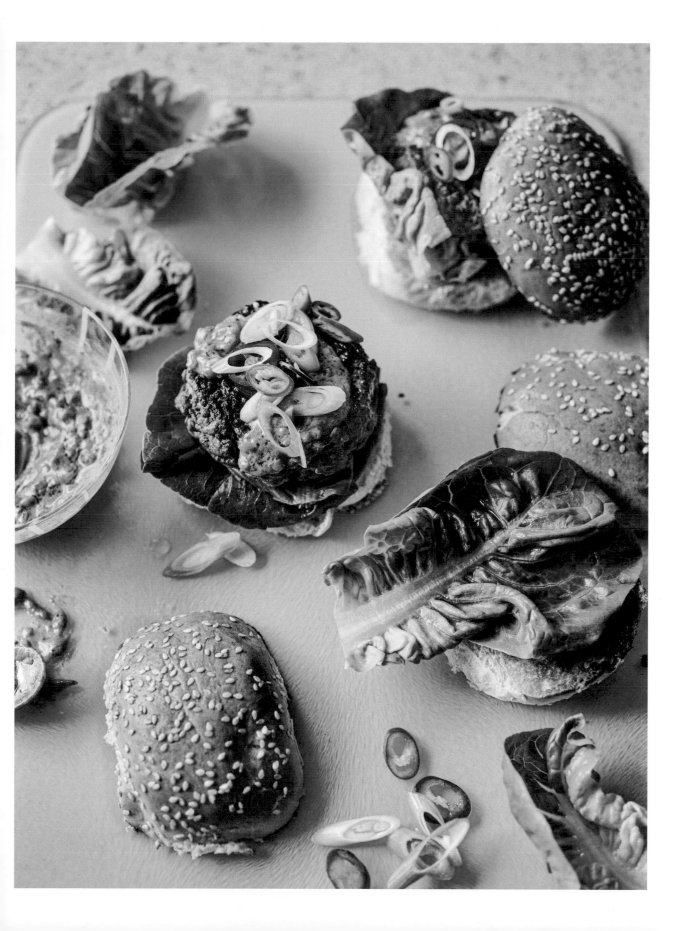

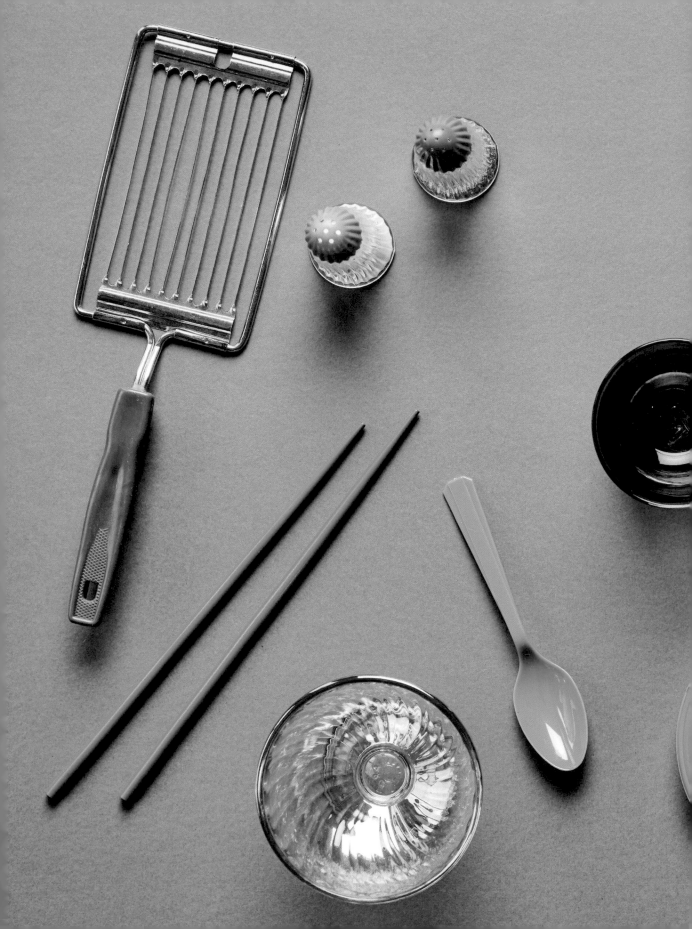

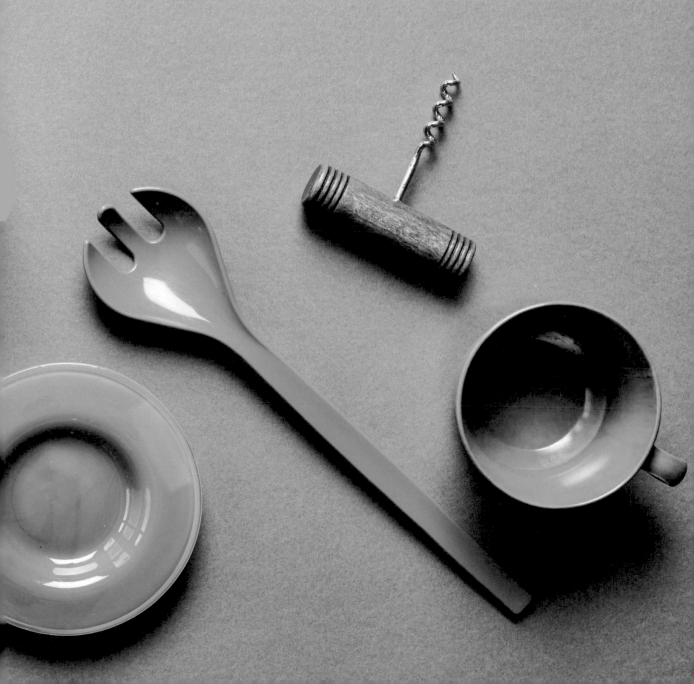

A BIT ON THE SIDE

• • • • • •

SALT & PEPPER CHIPS

Serves 4
272 calories

Salt and pepper chips is one of those side dishes that just begs to be eaten and enjoyed. There are certainly plenty of recipes out there for 'healthy' takes, but they use nonsense like MSG or sweetener in their ingredients, and there's just no need. The last thing we want to be doing when we're cooking is popping a chemical suit on. Don't get us wrong – MSG has its place and there's nothing wrong with it per se, but we prefer to make our taste from the ingredients in the dish.

This is one of those recipes that, if you have an air fryer to hand, can be prepped and cooked with absolute minimal effort. Air fryers have moved on from the dark days when they used to be the size of a tumble drier and resemble a helmet from a Daft Punk video. We're not ones for recommending fancy gadgets in the kitchen but we will cheerfully make an exception for these. That said, if you don't have one to hand or the counter space to allow one into the kitchen, fret not: you can just as easily make these in the oven.

This dish pairs nicely with the date-wrecking garlic beef (see page 133), although it reigns supreme when paired with a good chow mein.

1kg (2lb 3oz) potatoes, cut into chips (but not peeled)
2 tablespoons Worcestershire sauce
1 large onion, diced
1 red and 1 green chilli, finely sliced
1 teaspoon sugar
2 teaspoons salt
2 teaspoons five-spice
2 teaspoons chilli flakes

If you have an air fryer, pop everything in together and set it away until the chips are cooked. If not, preheat the oven to 200°C fan/425°F/gas mark 7. Tumble the chips around in the Worcestershire sauce and then bake in the oven for 30 minutes, or until cooked.

While the chips are cooking, spray a frying pan with a little oil and add the onion and chillies, cooking them over a medium heat until the onions have turned translucent.

Add the sugar, salt, five-spice and chilli flakes and stir.

Add the cooked chips and serve, basking in the glory of your creation.

Note from Paul
Cutting up chips can be an absolute ball-ache – do a giant batch and freeze half. If you are freezing uncooked chips, blanch them first – drop them into boiling water and boil for about 5 minutes, then put them into cold water, dry them off and bag them up.

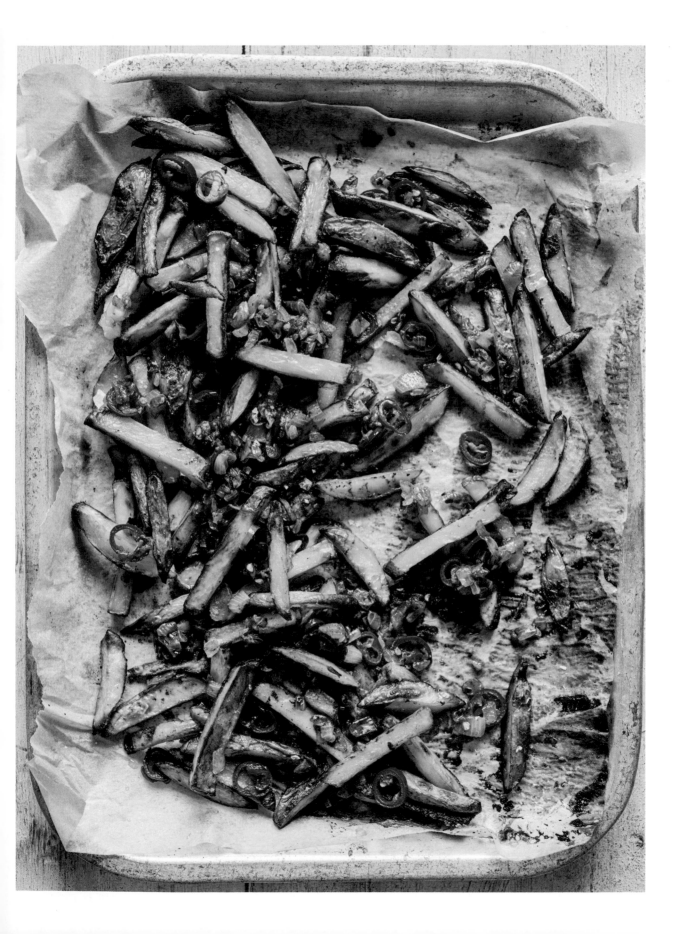

FIVE THINGS TO DO WITH A POTATO

1 medium potato
per serving

282 calories

I'm a huge fan of the humble potato: I just think they're neat. We have a tonne of recipes on the blog where we dice them, boil them, make cruel jokes about how Paul looks like a potato, and cover them in cheese. But sometimes the basics need looking at, so here are five basic tips for you to make the most of your potato when you're losing weight.

Oh – if you're someone who puts their Lidl shopping in a Waitrose bag so the neighbours think you're posh (we joke, but we know of at least two people who do exactly this), you can always swap out for a sweet potato. General rule of thumb for sweet potatoes is that they'll need a little less time in the oven – overcook them and you run the risk of pulling something out that looks like a collapsed lung. Caution!

Tiny anecdote for you now. I always remember boarding a flight and being lucky enough to have enough Air Miles for first class. I spent two weeks agonizing over whether I'd be accepted in my supermarket shoes and inevitably gravy-stained T-shirts, though I needn't have worried. The accolade for biggest knob on that flight went to the walking beetroot who, when the flight attendant offered to hang his jacket for him, haughtily replied, 'I think you'll find potatoes have jackets – this, madam, is a coat.' She had the good grace not to respond by tumbling him out of the exit doors, but I was so horrified by his snottiness and manner of talking to people that it was all I could do not to heartily break wind every single time I walked past his seat on the way to the toilet. What-am-I-like?

SEASONED WEDGES

Slice each potato in half (or into thirds if it's a particularly girthy beast). Then slice each half again, into wedge shapes. Tumble them around in a bowl with a few sprays of olive oil and whatever seasoning you fancy.

Spread them on a baking tray and cook at 200°C fan/425°F/gas mark 7 until they're crunchy (about 35–40 minutes). For the best wedges, whack them into an air fryer – less oil, better coverage.

For wedges, our favourite is a spoonful of olive oil and a beef stock cube crumbled on – trust us, it works!

PERFECT MASH EVERY TIME

154 calories

Never peel your potatoes, it's terrifically unnecessary and means you don't need to waste your life if you're left-handed like me and everything is a chore. Cut them into decent-size chunks and boil until they're soft enough to slide off a knife.

Drain off the water and tip them back into the pan together with a good pinch of salt and pepper. Crack an egg straight in and mash the hell out of everything.

If we may offer a further tip: buy a potato ricer – possibly one of the best 'gadgets' we use, for perfect creamy mash.

SIMPLE HASH BROWNS

198 calories

Grate a potato and an onion, using a coarse cheese grater.

Tip everything into a clean tea towel, mix in some salt and pepper, and squeeze every last bit of moisture out of the mixture – to be technical, you want it drier than a camel's urethra.

Squeeze the mix down into the oiled wells of a muffin tin and bake until crunchy, or fry in a few sprays of oil.

JACKET POTATOES

254 calories

Stab the potatoes all over with a sharp knife, or a fork if you're as cack-handed as Paul. Rub olive oil all over their skins – you don't need a lot. Sprinkle with salt and bake in the oven at 200°C fan/425°F/gas mark 7 until they're cooked through (about 1 hour–1 hour 20 minutes).

Once ready, score a cross on the top and pinch it apart, then top with all sorts of wonderful things – have a look on the blog if you're after some ideas!

LOADED POTATOES

427 calories

Cook the potatoes as above, but remove them from the oven about 10 minutes before they're done. Cut the potatoes in half and carefully scoop out the potato flesh and tip it into a bowl, leaving the skins intact. Mix in anything you like – cooked bacon, mature cheese and spring onion is our favourite.

Load the potato skins back up with the filling and pop them back into the oven until the tops are browned and everything looks spit-spot.

PINEAPPLE FRIED RICE

Serves 4
316 calories

1 onion, finely diced
4 cloves of garlic, finely chopped
½ teaspoon crushed chilli flakes
40ml (1½fl oz/3 tablespoons)
    chicken stock
1 egg
1 small carrot, grated
80g (3oz/½ cup) frozen peas
700g (1lb 9oz/3½ cups) cooked
    rice
    (see notes)
1 small tin of pineapple chunks,
    drained and roughly chopped
    into smaller chunks
2 tablespoons soy sauce
2 teaspoons fish sauce
2 teaspoons curry powder
juice of ½ a lime
3 spring onions, finely sliced
a handful of fresh coriander
    leaves

This recipe came about thanks to the success of two other recipes from our blog: our bacon and egg fried rice and our Hawaiian pizza pasta bake. This is handy for using up leftover rice and any stray tins of pineapple you may have hanging around.

This is another one you need to add to the 'hangover' list because it tastes even better the next morning, microwaved in a cereal bowl as you're hunched over your phone making sure you didn't upset anyone or send any angry texts to an ex. Add a load of soy sauce if you're feeling especially in need of a sodium bomb and a taste explosion. Make sure you reheat the hell out of it though: leftover rice is a volatile business, and we don't want to be held to account for any time you spend sitting on the toilet.

Place a large frying pan over a medium-high heat and spray with a little oil. Add the onion, garlic and chilli flakes and fry for about a minute, splashing in a little of the stock if starting to catch.

Crack the egg into the pan and stir quickly to scramble. Add the carrot and peas and cook for a further 1–2 minutes, adding the rest of the stock.

Add the rice and pineapple to the pan, then add the soy and fish sauces and the curry powder. Keep frying for 7–8 minutes, until the rice starts to crackle.

Remove from the heat and squeeze over the lime juice. Sprinkle over the spring onions and coriander leaves, and serve.

Notes from Paul
- *Cooked rice always works best when making fried rice, but if you don't have any to hand the microwave pouches will work fine.*
- *Leave out the fish sauce if you're not a fan – just add another tablespoon of soy sauce to compensate.*

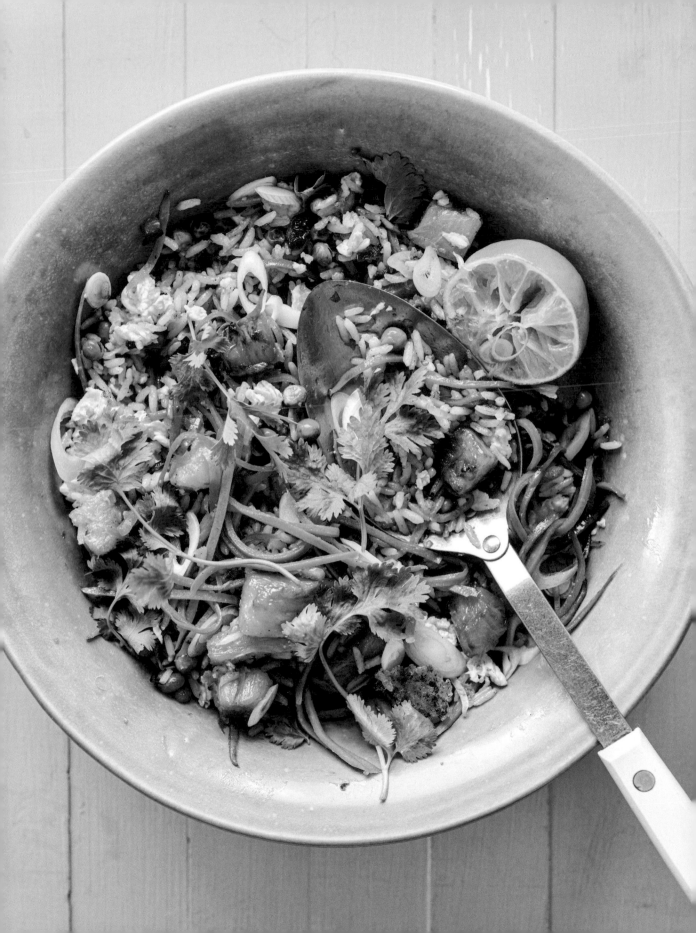

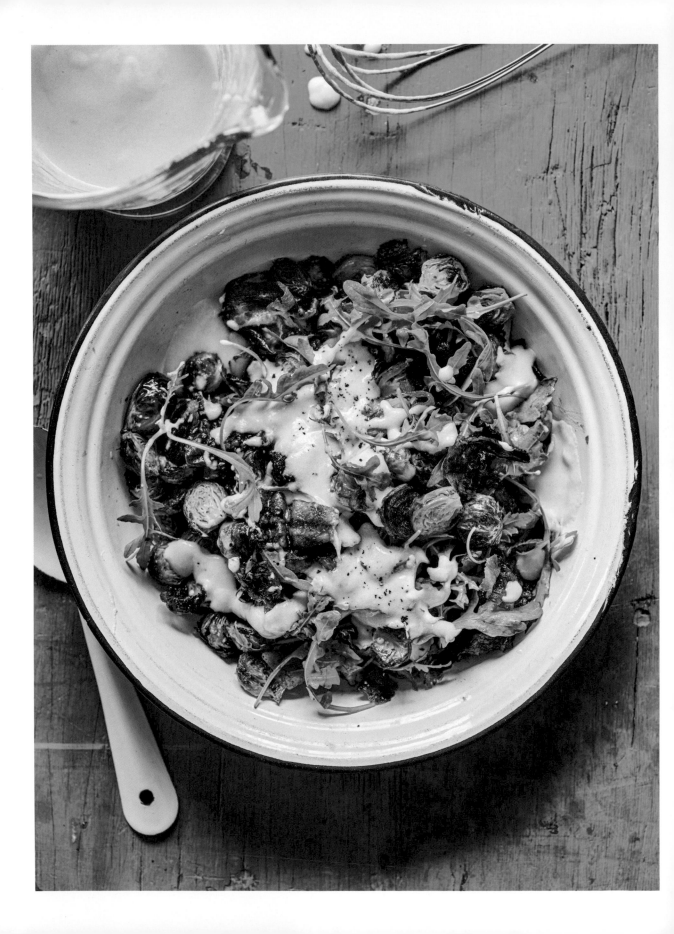

BACON & ROASTED SPROUTS WITH A CREAMY GARLIC SAUCE

Serves 4
370 calories

600g (1lb 5oz) sprouts
2 tablespoons olive oil
a pinch of sea salt
1 bulb of garlic
130g (4½oz) pancetta
300ml (10fl oz/1¼ cups)
    skimmed milk
1 heaped tablespoon plain flour
50g (1¾oz/⅓ cup) Cheddar
    cheese, the strongest you can
    find, grated
a couple of handfuls of rocket

Adding bacon to sprouts is common as muck these days, but we happened across this recipe while drinking our way around Banff and it's stuck with us ever since. Not least because the combination of sprouts and garlic has meant everyone within a forty-foot radius still visibly blanches every time we yawn.

Don't be put off by the humble sprout – yes, it's a little fart cushion, but if you've been put off by your nana boiling her Christmas sprouts since the summer solstice, you've never tasted them at their best.

Making a proper cheese sauce will always be worth it, so we've included it in the recipe below, but should you be pushed for time or want to keep the fat content a little lower, have a look at Paul's notes. This makes enough for a substantial side dish for two, but you could easily up the ingredients and have it as a main.

Preheat the oven to 200°C fan/425°F/gas mark 7 and dig out a good non-stick baking tray.

To prepare the sprouts, give them a rinse, remove any loose outer leaves, cut the stalks off the bottom, then slice in half. Pop the sprout halves (add the leaves too!) into a bowl, drizzle with the olive oil, add a pinch of salt, then tumble everything around so the sprouts get slick.

Cut the garlic bulb in half horizontally and rub any leftover oil and salt into the exposed cloves. Spread the sprouts over a baking tray, pop the garlic and pancetta into the gaps, and place in the oven to roast for around 25 minutes – you want the sprouts softened but still with a bit of crunch.

Five minutes before the sprouts are done, heat the milk in a pan and add the flour bit by bit, whisking as you go to avoid lumps. Then add the cheese and keep whisking until you have a thick sauce.

Take the sprouts out of the oven and squeeze a few of the softened garlic cloves into the sauce.

To serve, mix your rocket in with the warm sprouts and pancetta, and top with the sauce.

Notes from Paul
- *If you want to reduce the fat, use low-calorie spray and fat-free bacon (chopped).*
- *The cheese sauce is worth making, but if you're in a rush, use some low-fat cheese spread, thinned with milk, and mixed with the roasted garlic.*

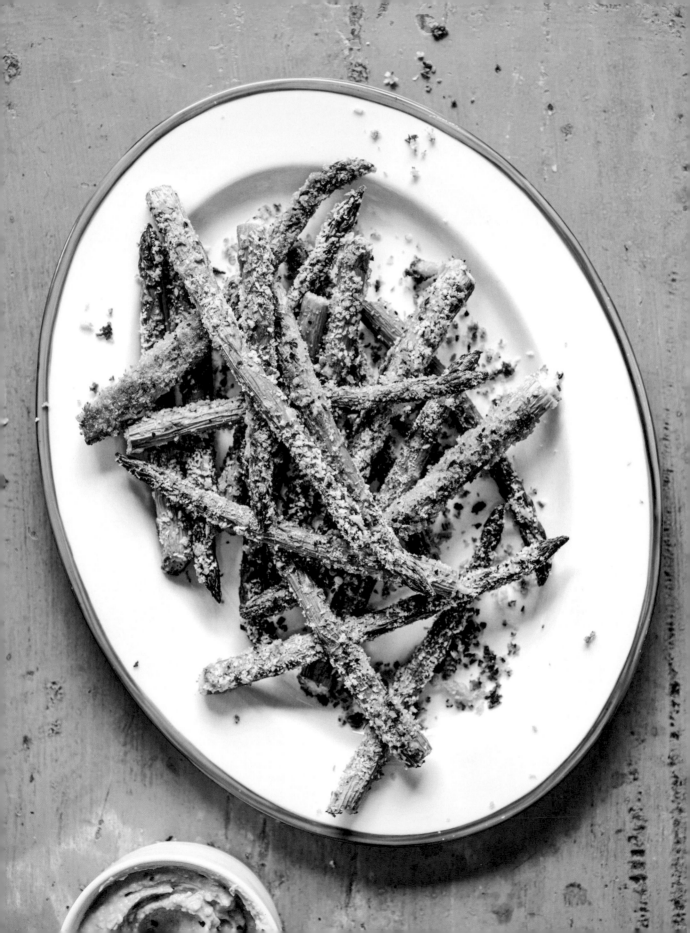

● ● ○ ● ● ●

CRISPY ASPARAGUS SPEARS

Serves 4
177 calories

70g (2½oz/⅔ cup) panko breadcrumbs
30g (1oz/¼ cup) grated Parmesan cheese
½ teaspoon crushed chilli flakes
2 eggs
500g (1lb 2oz) asparagus spears

You may be looking at these and thinking, well, why would you want asparagus spears? It's a fair question but please, let me explain. We wanted a recipe that was close to cheese straws – something quick to make and easy to dip. While looking for inspiration in the fridge, we spotted the same bunch of asparagus that we buy and replace every week, looking forlorn and miserable in the salad crisper drawer among all of the other 'good intention' vegetables we buy every week. It needed love, and I needed an excuse to holler from the bathroom that my wee smelled funny a few hours later, and so this recipe was born.

This is an excellent accompaniment to our Healthy Houmous on page 78. The breading and grilling recipe can be applied to all manner of vegetables, of course: try it with long strips of sweet red peppers, for example, or even some strips of carrot – though you may want to soften them up a little if you're not a fan of taking it raw. Always prep first.

Preheat the oven to 220°C fan/475°F/gas mark 9.

Combine the panko, Parmesan and chilli flakes in a shallow bowl. Beat the eggs well and pour into another shallow dish.

Dip each of the asparagus spears first into the egg, letting any excess dribble off, and then into the panko, making sure each spear is well coated. Place them on a baking sheet and spray with a little oil.

Bake for about 10 minutes, or until golden.

Notes from Paul
- These are great as a side, or as a snack.
- Add any herbs or spices you like to the panko mix – just be sure to mix them in well and ensure none have settled to the bottom of the bowl.
- You'll find panko in most supermarkets, but normal breadcrumbs will work too.

FIVE FABULOUS SIMPLE SIDES

●●●●●●

One of the most common questions we get asked via the blog, between folks sending us endless variations of 'I can't have potato, can you give me something to use instead of potato for your jacket potato recipe' nonsense, is 'what can I serve this dish with?' I used to answer eagerly, before the overwhelming lassitude that five years of writing brings me, but now I tend to reply with sarcasm. 'Disdain', I'll trill, or perhaps 'regrets', but it matters nought anyway – I could send a recipe for a medium-rare barbequed sofa cushion and I'd still get 'k thx hun xoxoxox' as a reply.

However, you have bought this book, and for that we love you dearly, so please find five quick recipes for sides – something a little extra you can serve with many of the recipes in this book. We tend to shy away from recommending that you must serve 'this' with 'that' because, why must you? Why must a burger always be with chips? Why limit yourself?

Oh, and as for the Bulgur Wheat Salad – we're big fans of throwing in cubed ham and feta together with some olives and strips of red pepper. Nothing fancy, no, but very easy to turn that one into a full lunch. Enjoy!

Serves 2
271 calories

PERFECT COLESLAW

Slice 1 red onion and ½ a red cabbage, and julienne 4 carrots. Whack them into a bowl, and stir in 5 tablespoons of yoghurt and 1 tablespoon of tahini.

Serves 4
236 calories

CREAMY CHEESY GREEN VEG MEDLEY

Chop up a head of broccoli and a head of cauliflower, throw in a good handful of quartered sprouts and slice a leek. Tip them all into a big saucepan with a bit of water and lightly steam until they soften but are still a bit firm.

Drain the veg and tip them into an ovenproof dish. Mix in 100g (3½oz/½ cup) of Philadelphia and a matchbox-size lump of grated Cheddar, and finally add a dash of salt and pepper. Pop under the grill for 10 minutes.

CREAMY SPINACH DIP

Serves 2
124 calories

Cook 600g (1lb 5oz) of frozen, chopped spinach according to the instructions. Drain well, allow to cool a bit, then squeeze every last drop of moisture out of it. Mix in 125g (4½oz/⅔ cup) of fat-free yoghurt and some sliced spring onions.

SORT OF MACHO PEAS

Get 3 big handfuls of frozen peas and cook them until softened. In a frying pan, gently cook a sliced onion. Chop up some mint and a chilli, and mix with the onions.

Drain the peas and chuck them into the pan, mash them a little bit with the back of a fork, add a small knob of butter, and mix together.

BULGUR WHEAT SALAD

Add 85g (3oz/½ cup) of bulgur wheat per person to a pan of boiling water, then crumble in a stock cube to add a bit of flavour. Cover the pan with a lid, reduce the heat and simmer for 15 minutes.

Gently fry a chopped onion in a pan and add some grated ginger, chopped mushrooms, a handful of frozen peas and some cubed carrots. Add some sliced peppers and cook until softened. Drain the bulgur wheat, add it to the pan of vegetables and stir well.

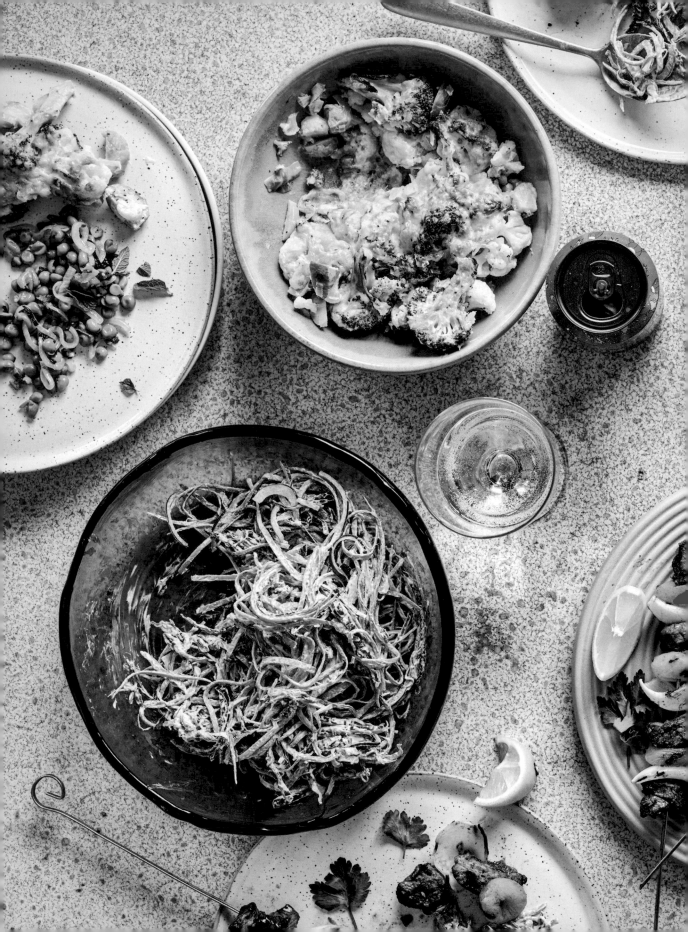

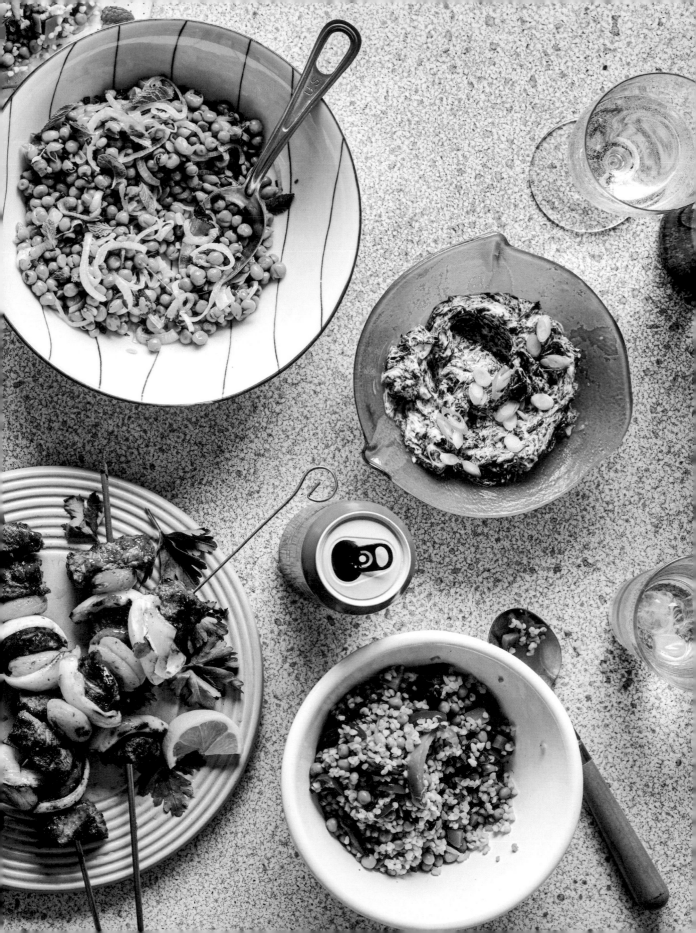

THREE QUICK DRINKS

Each drink serves 1

Drinks? In a cookery book? I hear your concerns and note them intently, but hear me out: the worst part for me about being on a diet in the middle of summer is not being able to have all the fancy-dan limited-edition drinks that the various fast food and coffee outlets release. I appreciate that some people have it worse off, yes, but is it really summer unless you've slipped into a sugar-coma thanks to your bucket of luridly-coloured fruit syrup? No.

So, please accept these drinks as the necessary compromises that they are and note that they serve a dual purpose alongside being delicious – they'll really knock the sweet tooth craving on the head. Give them a try and know this: we won't tell a soul if you happen to slip a little alcohol in there. We'd prefer you to do that here than in your breakfast smoothie.

180 calories

RASPBERRY ICE COOLER (opposite)

2 tablespoons sugar-free raspberry syrup
300ml (10fl oz/1¼ cups) skimmed milk
1 teaspoon sugar
1 tablespoon custard powder
½ teaspoon vanilla extract
6–7 large ice cubes

Drizzle 1 tablespoon of the raspberry syrup around the inside of the glass. Put everything else into a blender and blend, then pour!

64 calories

CARAMEL ICED COFFEE (see page 216)

200ml (7fl oz/¾ cup) brewed coffee, cold
1 teaspoon sugar
125ml (4fl oz/½ cup) unsweetened almond milk
6–7 large ice cubes
1 tablespoon sugar-free caramel syrup

Put everything into a blender and blend, then pour!

280 calories

WATERMELON AGUA FRESCA (see page 217)

¼ of a watermelon, cubed
juice of 1 lime
125ml (4fl oz/½ cup) cold water
2 teaspoons honey
ice cubes

Chuck everything into a blender and blend, then pour!

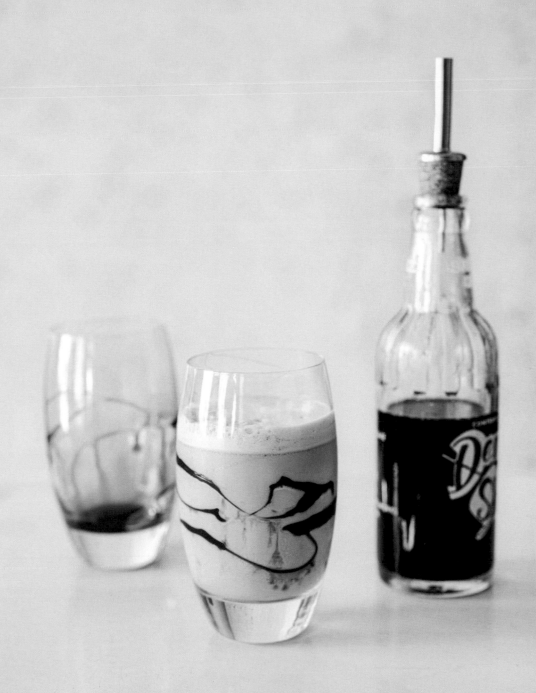

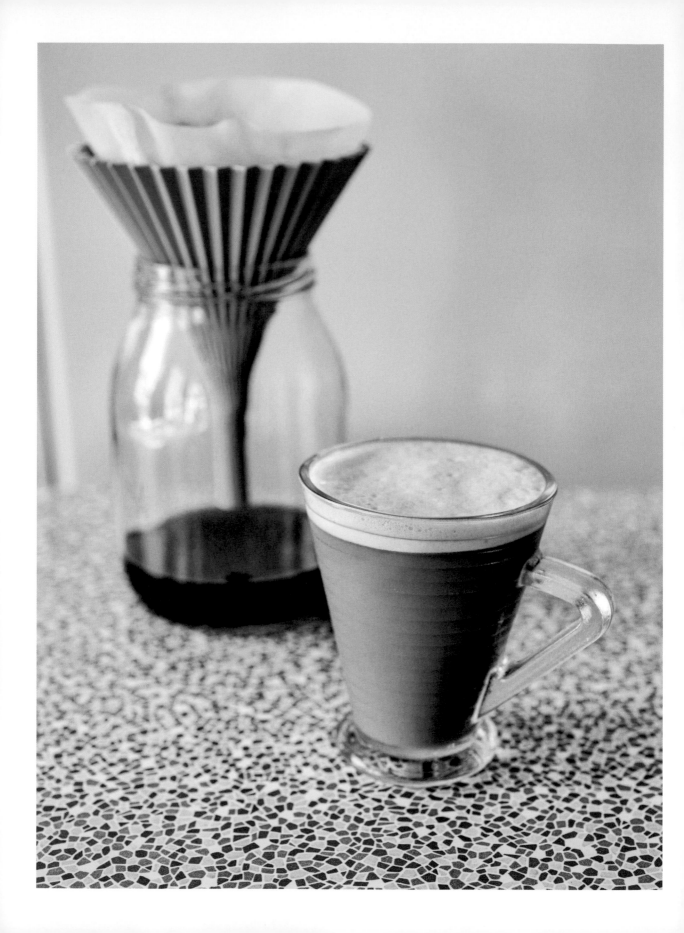

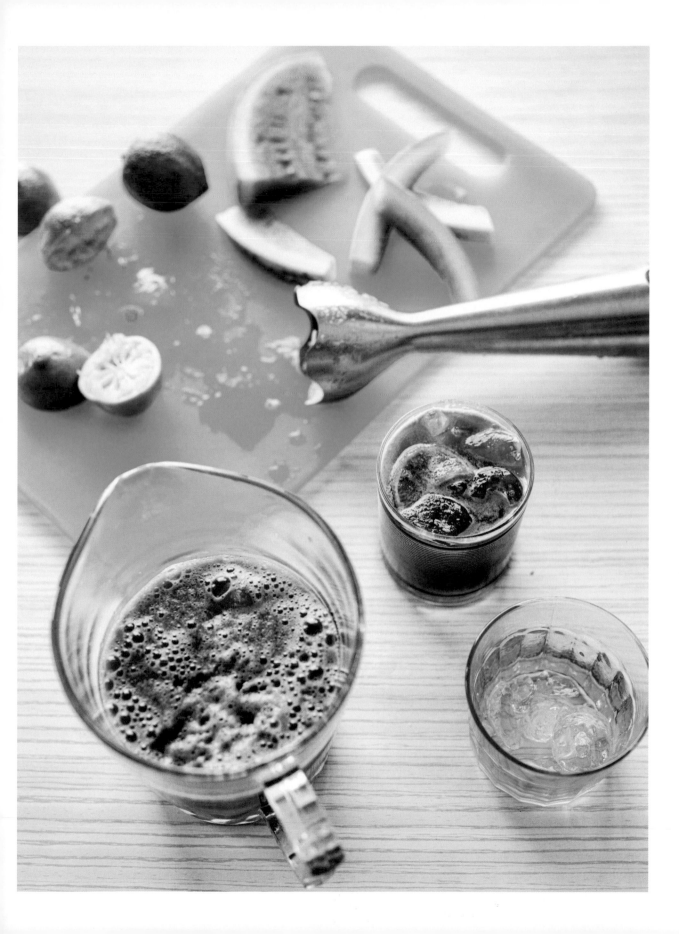

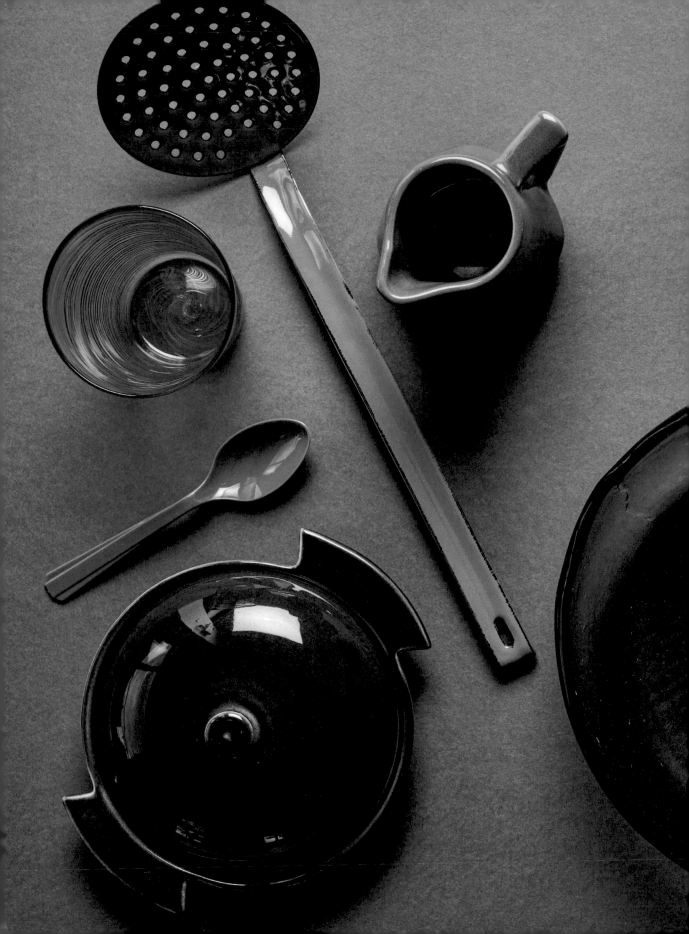

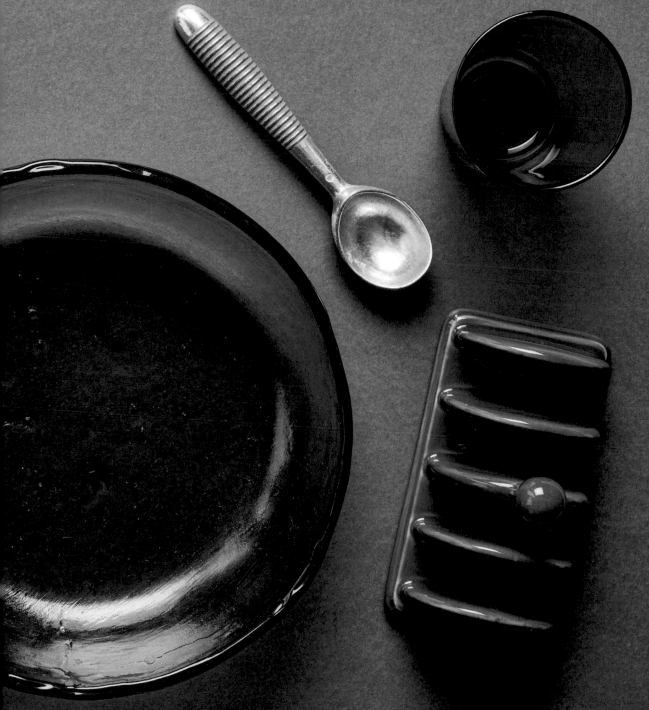

TREAT
YOURSELF

CHERRY BAKEWELL CHEESECAKE SHOTS

Serves 4
137 calories

We haven't been to many weddings as a couple – possibly because they don't want the headache of trying to work out whether to budget for six people on the catering front when we come blundering in, or maybe because we're intensely antisocial. Who can say? Well not us, because we don't want to talk to you.

However, our most recent wedding attendance inspired this recipe. We were served little shots of something sweet in between courses – presumably to amuse our bouches – and thus we took that idea and ran with it.

You can make any number of these small, luscious little desserts and then guiltily eat by the fridge while no one but your own pallid reflection judges you. They can be very easily slimmed down by using quark but why not make them as we intended and enjoy a small moment of pleasure instead?

Flavour these all sorts of different ways – stew some rhubarb and mix that through, or tip the layers the other way with some stewed apple and cinnamon at the bottom. Call it an apple crumble shot and goodness me, you'll barely keep folks from the door.

4 digestive biscuits
100g (3½oz/½ cup) extra-light soft cheese
100g (3½oz/½ cup) fat-free Greek-style yoghurt
a few drops of almond extract
1 small tin of cherries in juice

Get together some fancy long shot glasses if you have them, or swap them out for wee ramekins.

Crush up your biscuits (in your old tin can) and line the bottom of each glass.

Mix together the cheese, yoghurt and almond extract.

Before spooning the mixture on to the biscuit crumbs, take some of the juice from the cherries and swirl it through – don't aim to turn the whole lot pink, but to have some nice swirly-doos through the mix.

Spoon it on, and top with the cherries.

Note from Paul
If you find the yoghurt a little tart, add a teaspoon or 2 of icing sugar – we would normally recommend honey in this situation, but the flavour will clash with the almond.

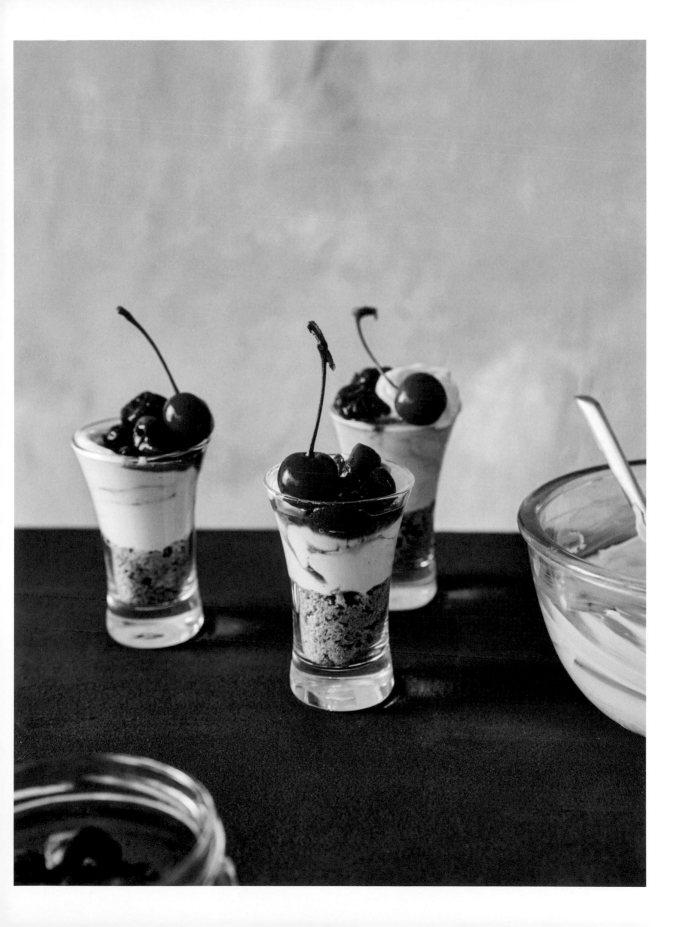

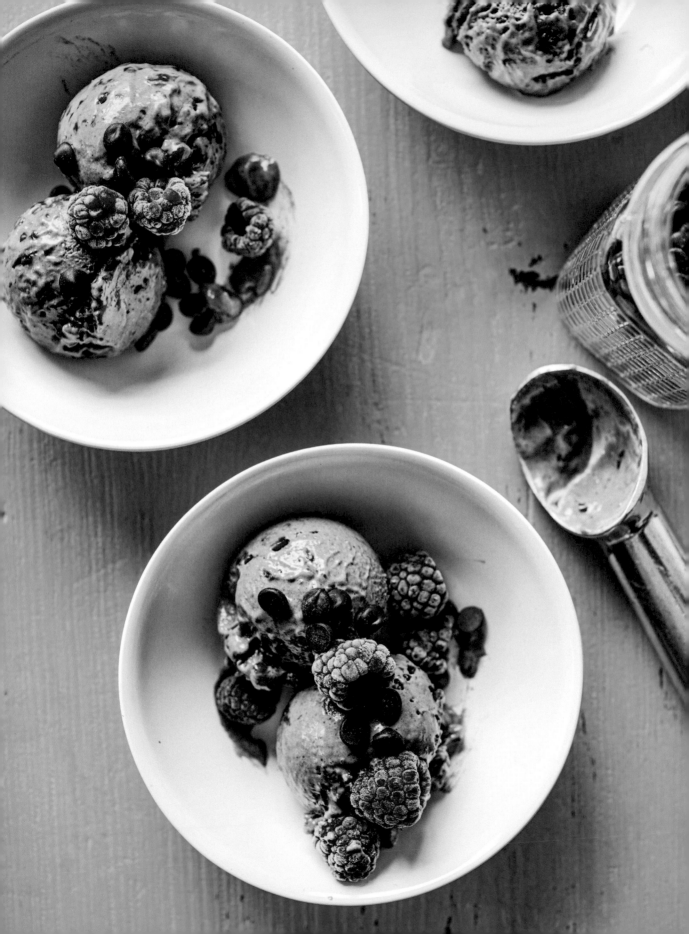

• • • • • •

DARK CHOCOLATE
AND RASPBERRY
ICE CREAM

Serves 4
134 calories

Listen. Nobody is going to pretend that you can sit eating your own weight in ice cream and get away with it on a diet. Everything in moderation, of course, but if you're anything like us, you can't have ice cream in the house without it beating away in the freezer like The Telltale Heart. I'm not saying I'm fat, but I have been known to drive home from the weekly shop balancing a tub of Häagen-Dazs between quivering thighs and scooping it up with lusty fingers. Embarrassing indeed.

Some 'slimming plans' will tell you that blending banana is the worst thing you can possibly do and you'll stay fat for ever more if you indulge in such frippery – we politely stick our fingers up at that notion. Of course, we encourage you to follow the rules to the letter but honestly, sometimes, just take a look at the logic.

This recipe is another that is infinitely customizable (Paul's added a few suggestions in the notes) – blend your banana, add your peanut butter (and you can leave that out if you're being terribly virtuous) and add what you like. The only thing to remember: you'll need frozen banana chunks. So, get into the habit of slicing up the brown bananas in your fruit bowl and freezing the segments so you're ready to go.

This recipe makes enough for two and is best eaten straight away without a moment of pause. Well, no, take it out of the blender first, we don't want you cutting that tongue of yours.

3 ripe bananas, cut into chunks and frozen
a good dollop of peanut butter
1 teaspoon good cocoa powder
a dribble of milk, should you need to thin it
a handful of frozen raspberries, plus extra to garnish
chocolate chips, to garnish

You'll need a good blender for this – something with a bit of zip. One of those wee stick blenders that couldn't cut tension won't do it.

Take a guess at what is next – we'll give you 10 minutes while we shuffle our shoes.

Blend the bananas with the peanut butter and cocoa powder.

Now – it won't look creamy right away, but bear with … keep your finger down on that blender … it'll suddenly look amazing, but if you like it a little thinner, add the milk.

Add the frozen raspberries and pulse a few times to combine – you don't want to blend them completely.

Serve sprinkled with extra frozen raspberries and chocolate chips.

Notes from Paul
- *Add mint if you fancy mint chocolate chip (who would have thought?!).*
- *Orange segments from a tin will make a tasty chocolate orange version.*
- *Skip the cocoa and add vanilla instead – and lo, what do you have?*

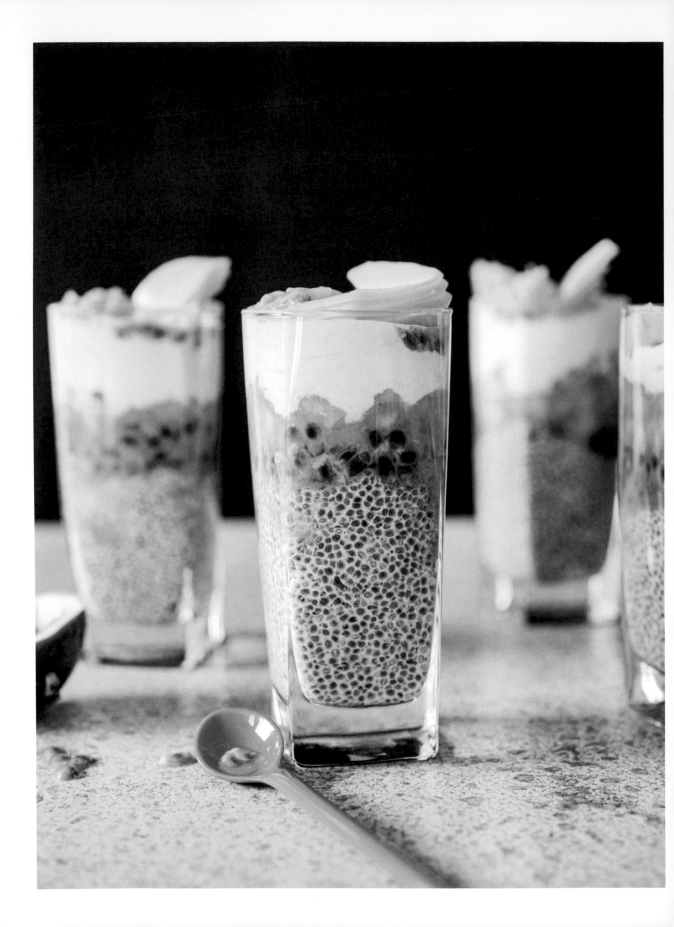

TROPICAL PARFAIT

Serves 4
210 calories

Confession time: we only learned what a parfait was from watching Shrek – any recipe that stems from words spoken by an animated donkey is bound to be a surefire hit. If you're common as muck, like us, you might think of this as a particularly fruity trifle, the same way I think of Paul. Well, he's certainly full of fat and jiggles when you shake him.

You mustn't let the thoughts of chia seeds put you off. For years we avoided them because I mean, take a look: they look like some awful frogspawn floating there. However, the chia seeds work really well in this and provide an interesting texture in what would be a bit of a plain-Jane dessert.

Don't be afraid to mix up your fruits – pretty much anything goes here, as long as you can take some of the juice and swirl it through. Actually, let me make a plea: expand your fruit repertoire! Paul used to be a right stinker when it came to trying anything new, preferring to stick to the hallowed apple, banana and orange trifecta learned in youth. Anything goes nowadays, so don't be afraid to mix it up!

85g (3oz/½ cup) chia seeds
500ml (18fl oz/2 cups) unsweetened almond milk
2 teaspoons vanilla extract
4 passion fruits, plus extra to decorate (optional)
275g (9¾oz/1½ cups) mango chunks, plus extra slices to decorate (optional)
250g (9oz/1¼ cups) fat-free natural yoghurt

In a bowl mix together the chia seeds, almond milk and vanilla extract.

Pour into 4 tall glasses or bowls and place in the fridge for 2 hours (or overnight).

Halve the passion fruits and scoop out the flesh into a bowl. Add the mango chunks and mash roughly with a fork.

Spoon the fruit mixture over the chia layer and top with the yoghurt.

Serve with extra mango slices and passion fruit on top, if using.

● ● ○ ● ● ●

CHOCOLATE MOUSSE

Serves 4
277 calories

Clutching your pearls, are you? The idea of a chocolate mousse setting your teeth all-a-clacker and making you think agitatedly of your waist? Don't – you're beautiful as you are, and anyway, we haven't steered you wrong yet. This is another dessert that serves up a decent mouth experience (yeah, I said it) while not being crazy high in fats and sugars.

We used to be served these mousses at school, although it's a safe bet to assume that neither chocolate nor anything approaching flavour had ever been mixed in. Never stopped me getting seconds, though (and this will be quite the revelation), as I was on good terms with the dinner lady. I'm assuming she saw a young lad with sagging boobs and a bumfluff 'tache and felt a connection.

This mousse can be livened up with either a little touch of peppermint essence and some tiny mint leaves stirred in, or, if you're feeling especially heroic, some chopped mandarin segments and a dewdrop of orange flavouring. Serve with a slice of cake the size of your head.

80g (3oz) milk chocolate
175ml (6fl oz/¾ cup) semi-skimmed milk
2 tablespoons honey
½ teaspoon vanilla extract
500g (1lb 2oz/2½ cups) low-fat Greek-style yoghurt
2 teaspoons icing sugar, to serve

Using a fine grater, grate all the chocolate into a bowl.

Pour the milk into a saucepan, then add the chocolate and very gently heat until it melts. Once the chocolate has melted into the milk, add the honey and vanilla and mix well.

Put the yoghurt into a large bowl and whisk well to incorporate some air into it. Gradually fold in the chocolate milk mixture, using a rubber spatula, and pour into individual bowls.

Chill in the fridge for 2 hours.

Before serving, sprinkle ½ teaspoon of icing sugar over each bowl.

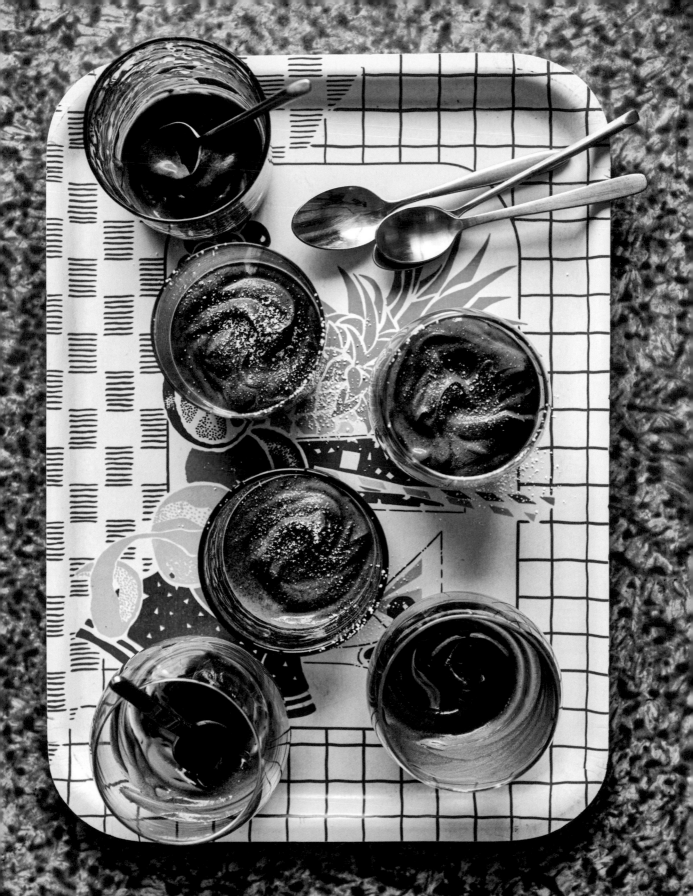

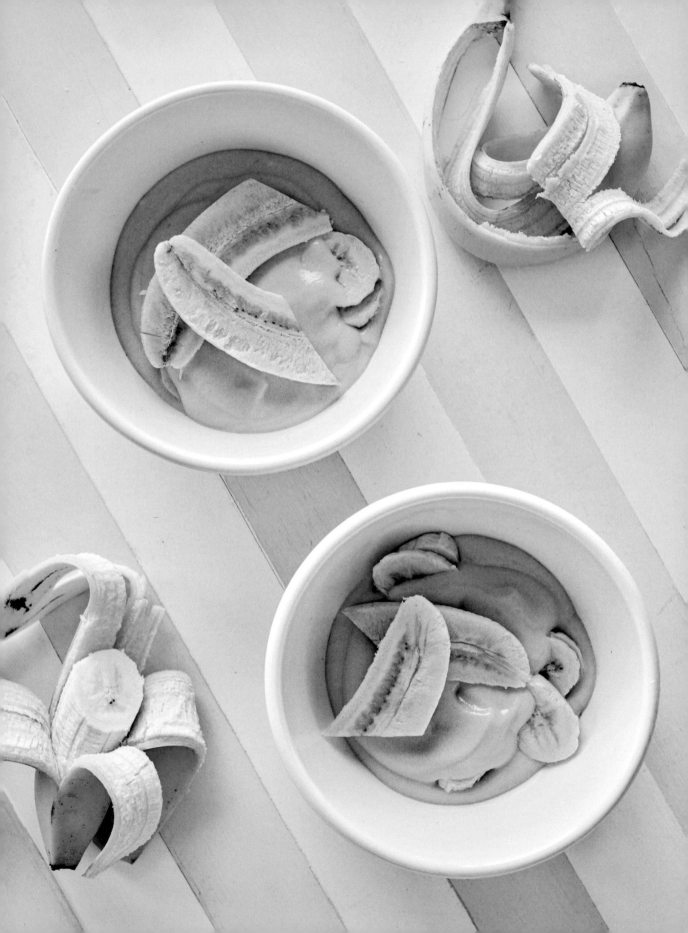

BANANAS & CUSTARD

•••••

Serves 4
308 calories

Bananas and custard are a meal from my childhood and although nostalgia can be a seductive liar, this is a dish I come back to time and time again. It's the type of dessert you can make for yourself and any little'uns you've got skedaddling around your ankles.

Speaking of children, we are often asked whether we have ever considered being parents: it usually takes about fifteen minutes for the hurt and ire to leave the questioner's face when I laugh out loud at their silly question. You have to understand that Paul and I can barely look after ourselves, never mind nine pounds of mewling poop machine. Plus, I've already got one bald bad-tempered, boggly-eyed attention drain, I don't require another.

Paul, on the other hand, is an absolute wonder with babies. When my sister gave birth to Jake, Paul was cooing at his cradle and making a fuss within seconds. Jake was transfixed, though I maintain it's because he took one look at Paul's expansive rack and thought he was set for life. As a result, Paul would love to father a child – we compromised and got a second cat.

If you're looking to gussy up this recipe, you could do worse than caramelizing the bananas – slice them into long halves, sprinkle on some brown sugar and grill them for a few minutes. Watch the top of your mouth on that boiling sugar though – if you're anything like us, the bananas won't make it to the bowl before you 'have a try'. Good luck!

500ml (18fl oz/2 cups)
    unsweetened almond milk
6 egg yolks
100g (3½oz/½ cup) sugar
2 tablespoons cornflour
1 teaspoon vanilla extract
4 bananas

Heat the almond milk in a saucepan until the edges are just starting to bubble – don't boil it!

In another bowl, whisk together the egg yolks, sugar and cornflour. Gently ladle the warmed milk into the egg mixture just a little at a time, whisking continuously.

Return the whole lot to the pan and cook over a medium-low heat, stirring constantly, until it coats the back of a spoon. Remove from the heat, add the vanilla extract and leave to cool in the fridge for about an hour or so.

Slice the bananas and stir into the mixture, keeping back a few slices for the top.

Notes from Paul
- *If you've got an ice cream maker this works brilliantly!*
- *Use any fruit you like – we used bananas because we had some left over, but anything will do!*
- *Swap out some of the sugar for sweetener if the amount is making you anxious, but don't replace the lot. Be aware it will likely be a bit thinner, but you can add a little more cornflour to counteract that.*

• • • • •

LEMON & LIME ROULADE

Serves 4
183 calories

2 large eggs
50g (1¾oz/¼ cup) caster sugar
50g (1¾oz/4 tablespoons)
   self-raising flour
150g (5½oz/¾ cup) quark
100g (3½oz/½ cup) fat-free
   Greek-style yoghurt
zest and juice of 2 lemons
zest and juice of 2 limes

So, we have a confession. We have always been about 'proper cooking' rather than making dismal desserts – but we have absolutely tried all the different permutations of cakes, nonsense and flimflam that get wheeled out as 'free' on certain diets. Readers, I've genuinely never wished for death harder than when someone baked me a roulade that they reassured me was 'just like the real thing', despite not having flour or sugar in it. It was like sucking the caretaker's mop from a haunted school. I remember her eyes brimming with joy, her whiskery lips a-tremble as I tried it, and I just didn't have the heart to tell her I've eaten tastier things from the depths of my chest hair. I reassured her it was 'just delicious', and she went on to spread that recipe far and wide. Perhaps I'm the cause of all those awful recipes.

The dilemma here is that we want to include a cake, but not a 'slimming' cake – just a good, light, easy to make dessert that you can have a small piece of, serve it with whatever you want and enjoy it. Remember: a little of what you fancy does you good. You might balk at the sugar and flour but overall, it's not too bad, and when filled to the brim with your creamy middle, it makes for a delicious dessert.

Preheat the oven to 180°C fan/400°F/gas mark 6 and line a Swiss roll tin with greaseproof paper.

Beat the eggs and sugar together until thick. Gently fold in the flour gradually and pour the mixture into the Swiss roll tin.

Bake in the oven for 10–12 minutes, until golden.

Meanwhile, mix together the quark and yoghurt along with the zest and juice of the lemons and limes.

Remove the sponge from the oven and allow to cool.

Once cool, spread the quark mixture over the top of the sponge, leaving a bit of space at the edges. Gently roll the sponge over itself to make the familiar Swiss roll shape, peeling away the greaseproof paper as you go.

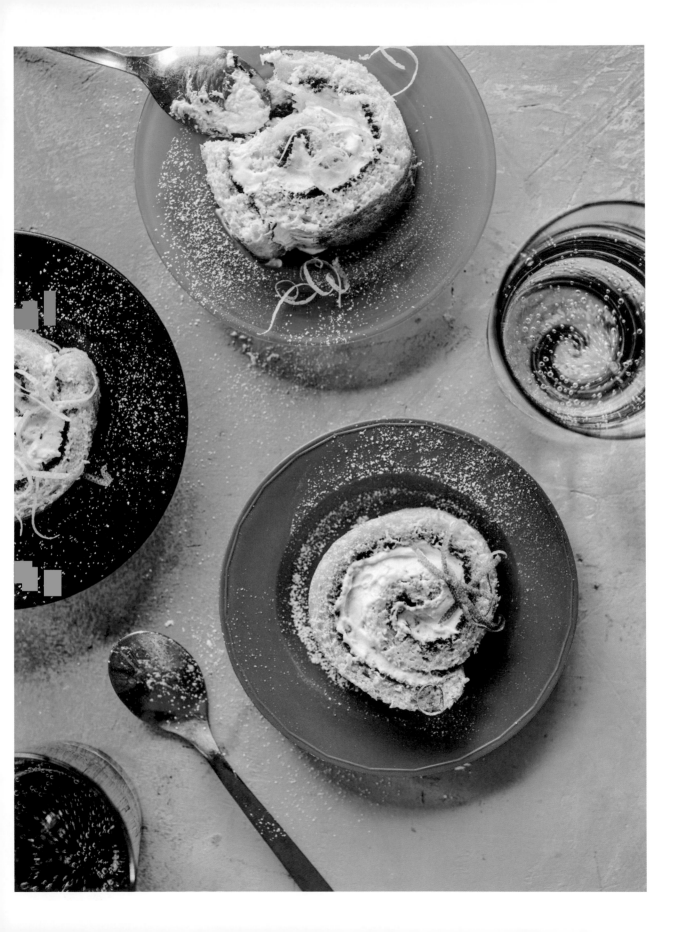

CHOCOLATE BANANA BREAD

Makes 8 slices
223 calories per slice

4 very ripe bananas, mashed, plus 1, halved lengthways, for decoration
2 eggs
50g (1¾oz/¼ cup) low-fat Greek-style yoghurt
2 tablespoons oil
2 tablespoons honey
1½ teaspoons vanilla extract
200g (7oz/1½ cups) wholewheat flour
30g (1oz/⅓ cup) cocoa powder
1 teaspoon ground cinnamon
a pinch of salt
1 teaspoon bicarbonate of soda
½ teaspoon baking powder
2 tablespoons chocolate chips

This recipe is a favourite of my sister – Deborah (and never Debra, mind you, and she will absolutely cut your face if you make that error) – and it seems only fitting that I reflect on growing up with her before we launch into the recipe. She did, after all, turn me into the man I am today: socially awkward, thoroughly bullied and interestingly scarred.

My sister is the literal antithesis of me: where I'm tall, she's short. Where I'm fat, she's stick thin (no matter what she eats: she remains the only person who can put away a family-size Dominos order and still disappear when she turns sideways). Whereas growing up I was cool, calm and collected, she was like a cat with a burning tail. Such anger. Not a day went by when we weren't shouting and screaming at one another, and things came to a terrifying head when she lobbed an entire DVD box set of 24 off my skull. I still see Kiefer Sutherland when I blink.

However, since moving out, absence has made the heart grow fonder and now we get along like a house on fire – on the one day a year that we are thrown together, under the guise of celebrating Christmas. It's been interesting watching the hellcat turn into a vision of domesticity, while I ever-so-slowly tumble in the other direction, and I know she will be delighted to see this little tribute in the book. In the copy that she's stolen from my mother, and is using to prop her front door open so she can smoke on the doorstep like the slattern she is.

Paul also has a sister.

Preheat the oven to 170°C fan/375°F/gas mark 5 and line a medium loaf tin with greaseproof paper.

Mix together the bananas, eggs, yoghurt, oil, honey and vanilla extract in a bowl until well combined.

Add the flour, cocoa powder, cinnamon, salt, bicarbonate of soda and baking powder and gently fold in until well mixed, but don't overdo it!

Pour the mixture into the lined loaf tin, sprinkle the chocolate chips over and top with the banana halves, cut-sides up. Bake for an hour, then test with a skewer to make sure it comes out clean – if it needs a bit longer, bake for another 5 minutes and test again.

Turn out on to a rack and allow to cool.

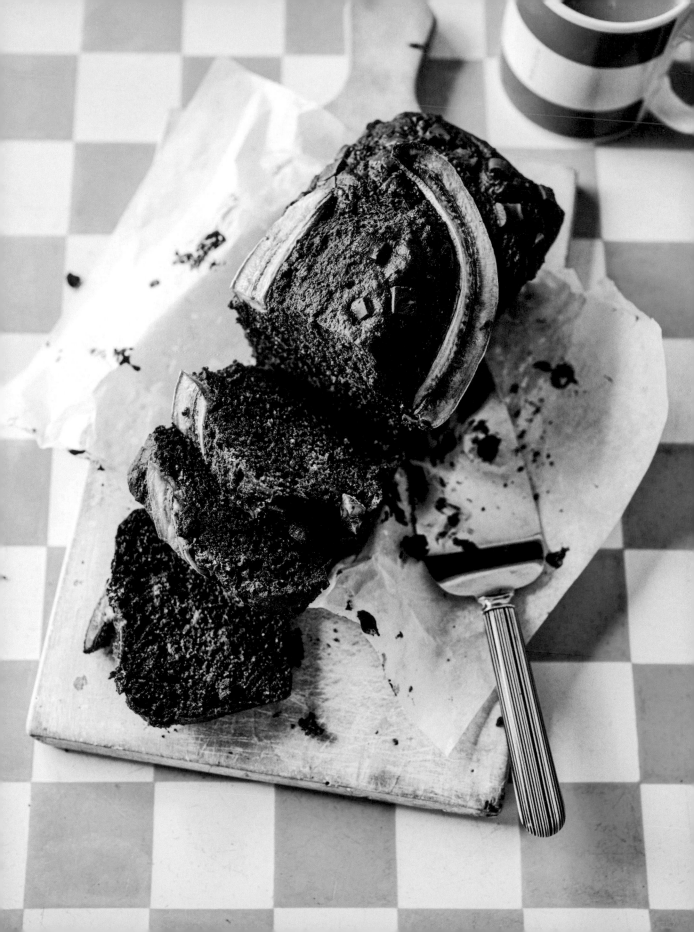

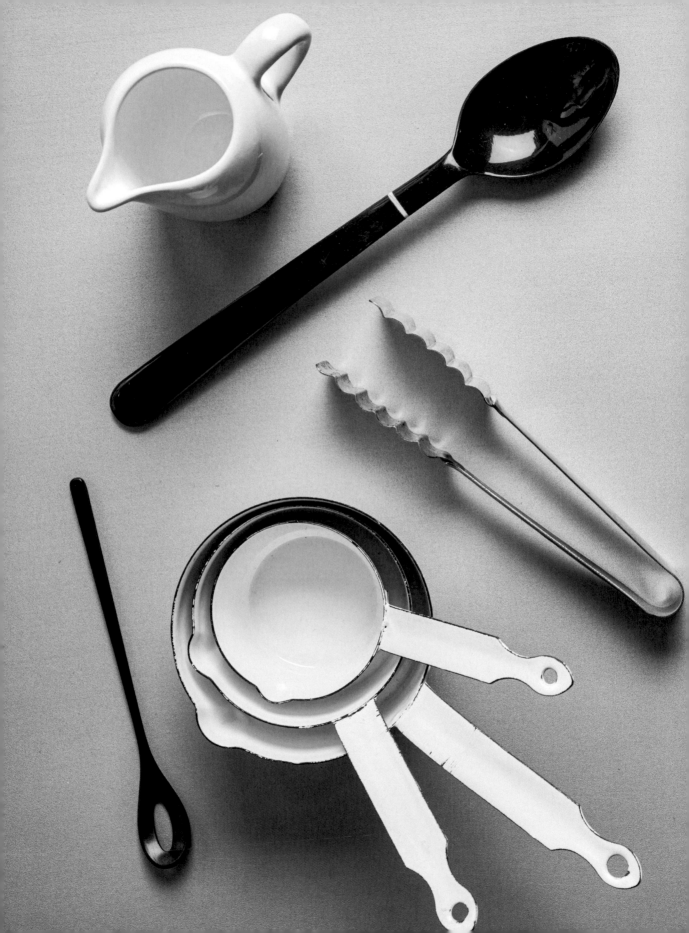

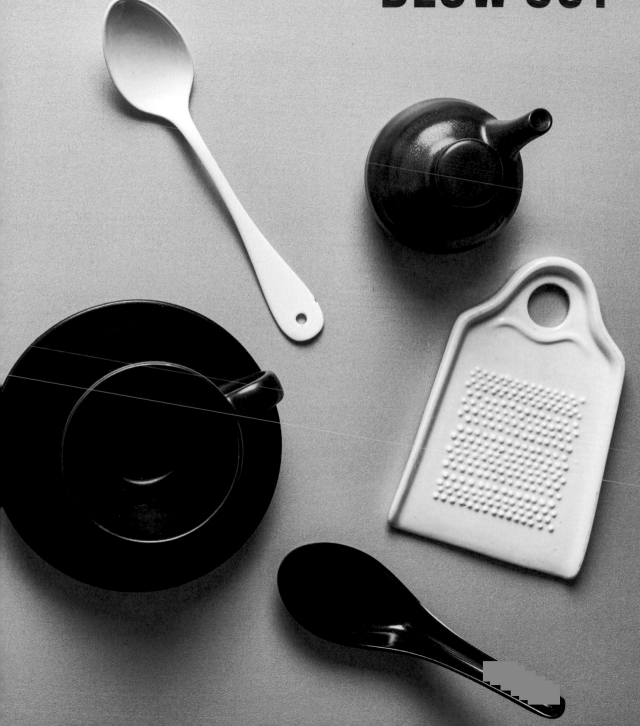

THE OCCASIONAL BLOW OUT

THE BEST CHILLI MACARONI CHEESE

● ● ● ● ● ●

Serves 6
946 calories

Macaroni cheese is my favourite meal. As a consequence, you can believe that we have tried every single variation you can think of when it comes to macaroni cheese: fried macaroni cheese balls were a highlight, but the winner has to be the dish we made with double cream and five separate cheeses. We added chorizo, lardons and chest pains, and lived like kings. We took a moment over how much damage we had done to our diet and found that we'd exceeded our weekly 'allowance' in just one bowl. But what a bowl!

We can't, in all good conscience, replicate that dish here. We're all for treating yourself, but we're also fairly sure that we don't want to be responsible for lots of gloomy face-ache shots of you all in the newspapers saying we've made your ankles swell. So, please, take this dish as the compromise between the pure sex that was the best macaroni cheese I've ever had and those awful 'slimming' dishes that get served up by people who have never known joy. It's delicious, but it absolutely won't wreck your week. Enjoy!

80g (3oz) butter
80g (3oz/⅔ cup) plain flour
1 teaspoon Dijon mustard
60ml (2fl oz/¼ cup) double cream
1 litre (1¾ pints/4 cups) whole milk
300g (10½oz/3 cups) mature Cheddar cheese, grated
1 teaspoon freshly ground black pepper
400g (14oz/3 cups) dried macaroni
100g (3½oz) bacon lardons
100g (3½oz) chorizo, diced
100g (3½oz) jalapeños, chopped
75g (2¾oz) sun-dried tomatoes, drained and finely chopped
50g (1¾oz/¾ cup) Parmesan cheese
50g (1¾oz/½ cup) panko breadcrumbs

Preheat the oven to 180°C fan/400°F/gas mark 6.

Melt the butter in a large saucepan, then stir in the flour and cook for 1 minute. Add the mustard and remove the pan from the heat.

Gradually whisk in the cream and the milk, then pop the pan back on the heat and cook gently, stirring constantly, until it starts boil and thickens.

Remove the pan from the heat, add the Cheddar, and stir until melted. Add the black pepper and stir well to combine.

Bring a large pan of salted water to the boil and add the macaroni. Simmer for 10 minutes, then drain.

Spray a small pan with a bit of oil and cook the lardons and chorizo until crisp.

Stir the macaroni into the cheese sauce along with the jalapeños, lardons, chorizo and sun-dried tomatoes. Tip into an ovenproof dish and sprinkle the panko and the Parmesan over the top.

Bake in the oven for 25–30 minutes.

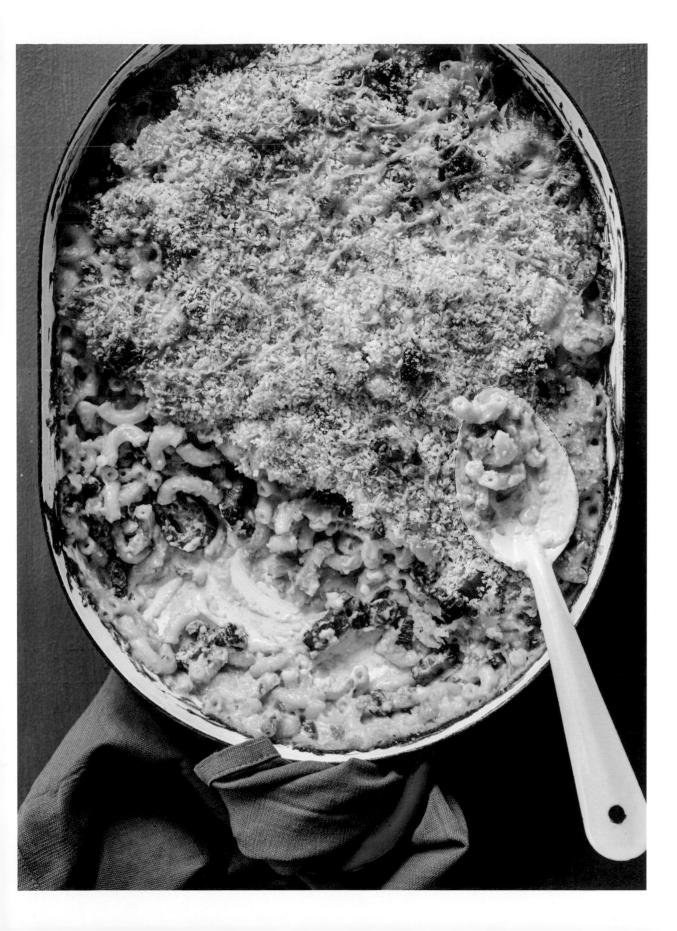

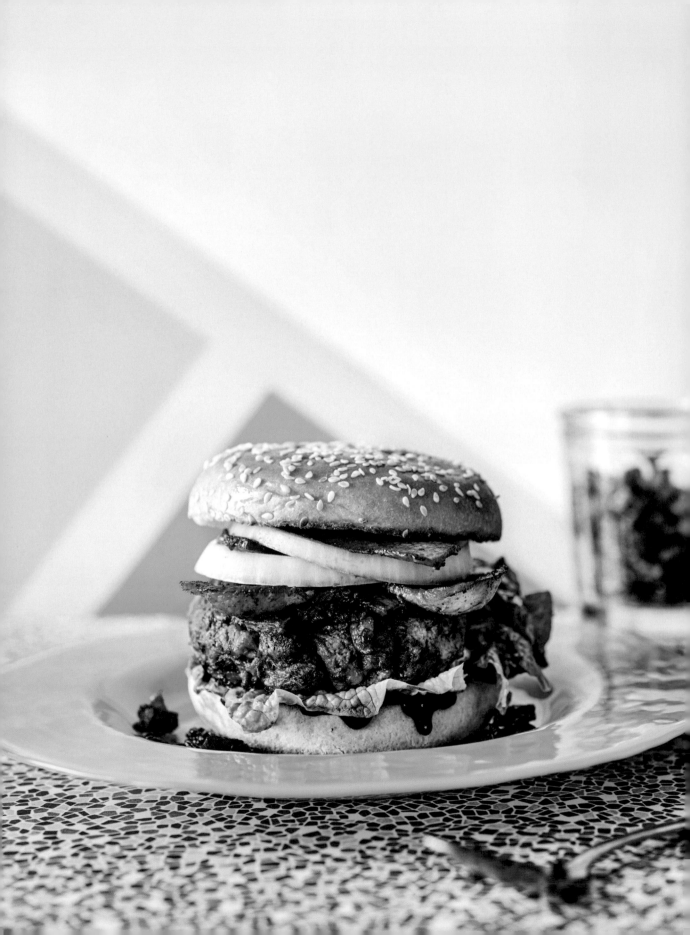

BACON JAM
BACON BURGER

Serves 4
696 calories

We were torn, so very badly, as to whether or not to put this bacon-three-way burger into the book. See, sticking bacon in everything seems like part of a phase the internet went through a few years ago.

We're always late to the party when it comes to fads and crazes. Building an online presence demands being at the cut-and-thrust of internet hilarity, and we fail miserably. I only participated in the planking craze because I was glad of a lie down and a chance to let my cankles drain. Paul went all-in on those 'charity wristbands' a few years ago and proudly sported a garish bangle to promote awareness of bad circulation, though that seemed a little remiss when the combination of his fat wrists and the unforgiving car-boot-quality elastic meant his fingertips went black.

And so it is with the bacon craze. But frankly, screw any concerns about this being old-hat: this burger tastes absolutely amazing and if you're going to give yourself a meaty mouthful, adding bacon is only ever going to raise the game.

For the burger
2 rashers of back bacon, diced into small cubes
4 rashers of streaky bacon
400g (14oz) beef mince
4 baps
4 tablespoons barbecue sauce
a handful of Cos lettuce
1 large onion, sliced

For the bacon jam
350g (12½oz) bacon medallions
2 large red onions, finely diced
2 tablespoons balsamic vinegar
2 tablespoons tomato sauce
salt and freshly ground black pepper

First, make the bacon jam by frying the bacon medallions until they're nice and crispy. Remove from the heat and chop to the same size as the finely diced onions.

Spray a pan with a little oil and add the red onions, chopped bacon, vinegar, tomato sauce, a pinch of salt and pepper and 4 tablespoons of water. Cook slowly and gently for about 30 minutes, stirring occasionally and adding a little more water or vinegar if it looks like it needs it, until the mixture has a jammy consistency.

To make the burgers, heat a large frying pan over a medium-high heat and add a little oil.

Add the diced bacon to the pan and fry until crisp. Scoop the bacon out of the pan and place onto a plate to cool for a few minutes.

Put the pan back over the heat and add the streaky bacon. Cook until crisp, then remove from the pan to another plate.

Put the mince and diced bacon into a bowl and mix well, but be careful not to over-mix. Divide the mix into 4 equal-sized balls and squash each one down into a rough burger shape.

Fry the burgers for 3–4 minutes on each side.

To assemble your burgers, cut each bap in half and spread the barbecue sauce over the bottom half. Follow with some lettuce, then the burger, then the bacon jam, the slices of streaky bacon, some onion and finish with the top half of the bap.

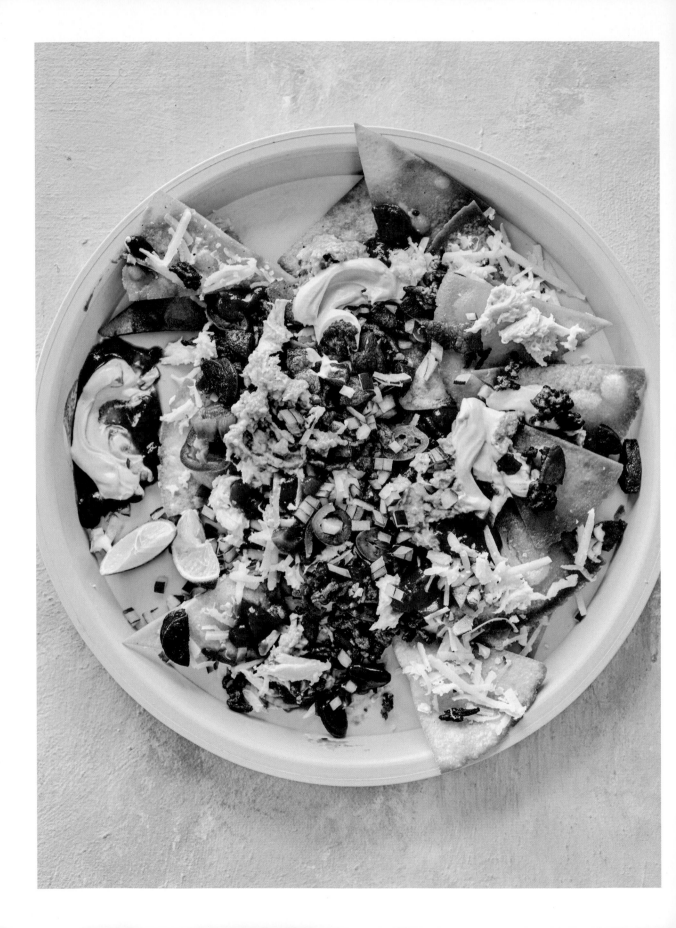

• • ○ • • •

HOMEMADE NACHOS

Serves 6
787 calories

The very best nachos we've ever had were in a tiny in-through-the-door-out-through-the-window bar outside Vancouver. The only thing I expected from this place was a glassing and an ambulance ride, but nevertheless, our stomachs pulled rank and we ordered the nachos off the menu behind the bar. What came out was a Sputnik-sized bowl of wonder: nachos topped with all sorts of different cheeses, a homemade chilli, gherkins and pickles and salsa and sour cream and guacamole and corned beef …

… and honestly, I've had to push my chair back a few inches just remembering that meal. If the Devil himself appeared and offered me a chance to go again on that dinner in exchange for Paul's life, I'd be ushering my beloved into the light before you could say, 'But I thought we were forever.' Poor lad, I'm being cruel – this recipe actually came about as a result of Paul trying to replicate that dish, and he's actually made a decent fist of it.

In absolutely no way is the recipe – as it is written – good for your diet if you're having it every day. But once in a while, give it a go. Of course, you could make a couple of swaps to make it healthier, if you positively must. We'll turn the other cheek.

250g (9oz) beef mince
100g (3½oz) chorizo, diced
4 rashers of bacon, diced
½ teaspoon garam masala
6 corn tortillas
2 litres (1¾ pints/4 cups) vegetable oil
1 × 400g (14oz) tin of spicy beans, drained of excess sauce
1 red onion, diced
350g (12oz/2½ cups) grated Cheddar cheese
100g (3½oz/½ cup) grated mozzarella
a handful of jalapeño peppers, sliced
4 tablespoons sour cream
4 tablespoons guacamole
4 tablespoons hot salsa

Heat a frying pan over a medium-high heat and add the beef mince, chorizo and bacon.

Fry until all the mince is browned and the bacon is crispy, then stir in the garam masala and set aside.

Slice the tortillas into nacho shapes – or whatever shape you like!

If you have a deep-fat fryer, heat it to 180°C(350°F), otherwise pour the oil into a large, heavy-bottomed saucepan and heat it over a medium-high heat.

Once the oil is at temperature, add the tortillas in small batches at a time – they're done when they're crispy and the surface is bubbled. Carefully remove each batch from the oil and drain on some kitchen paper, then continue frying the rest.

Once the nachos are cooked, tip them on to a large plate and top with the mince mixture. Sprinkle over all the other ingredients – don't be dainty, slop it all on there.

THE OCCASIONAL BLOW OUT

●●●●●●

CURRYWURST PICKERS

Serves 4
584 calories

This recipe lives and dies on the quality of your sausage, so don't be tempted to rush out and buy those awful pink cylinders full of bumholes and eyelids but instead, invest in good sausages. Even better, go down the proper German sausage route – you'll thank me later.

This recipe comes from our (albeit hazy) memories of our holiday in Berlin. Berlin's a fantastic place, full of easy eating and sleazy adventure, and it remains so much to my permanent chagrin that Paul won't let me move over there. Never has a city sung to me so beautifully as Berlin, and I feel as though I've only just scratched the surface of what it can do to me. Outside our hotel was a wonderful little stall selling currywurst. Just the thing to grab before a drunken stumble back to the room.

This recipe might seem like a bit of a hassle – making the sauce, making the potatoes – but Paul's included a couple of ways to speed it up in the notes. We apologise to each and every German who may be mortified by our cooking ability, but this is what we do.

Oh! These are just the thing for when your slimming club insists you bring along something for taster night: you can make them the night before, thoroughly enjoy every last one and bring along a punnet of scabby grapes like everyone else.

You can find our recipe for the best roast potatoes you'll ever eat on page 244, or, if you're watching your figure, simply cut up your potatoes, spray them with a little oil, crumble an Oxo cube over them and pop them into the oven. If you bake them along with the sausages, the fat from the sausages will make them crunchy.

16 roast potatoes (see page 244)
6 good-quality sausages

For the sauce
250g (9oz/1 cup) passata
1 tablespoon smoked paprika
1 teaspoon chipotle tabasco
    sauce
3 tablespoons curry powder, plus
    extra for sprinkling
2 tablespoons honey
2 tablespoons lemon juice

In a small pan, simmer all the sauce ingredients ever so slowly until you get a thick, smooth sauce.

Meanwhile, set about making your roasties and cooking your sausages however you fancy.

Once everything is cooked, pop the sauce into a dish (sprinkling with a touch more curry powder). Slice your sausages into thirds and skewer each chunk with a cocktail stick and a chunky roastie.

Enjoy, dipping into the sauce as you go

Note from Paul
If you can't be fussed making a fruity curry sauce, no problem – you can buy curried tomato sauce in the supermarket, or stir some curry powder into ketchup for a close enough alternative.

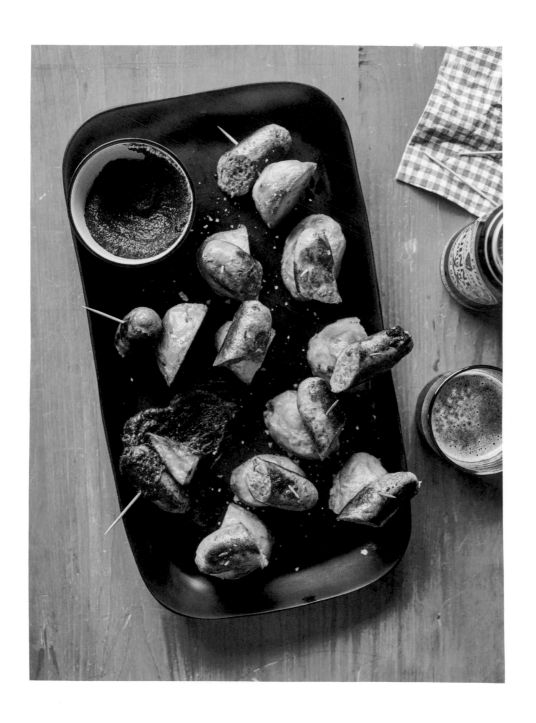

SOME HEATHENS (PAUL) LIKE MAYONNAISE ON TOP OF THE SAUCE, BUT DON'T LISTEN TO HIM, HIS EYES ARE TOO CLOSE TOGETHER TO BE TRUSTED.

EMOTIONAL SUPPORT POTATOES

Serves 1
604 calories

Maris Piper potatoes – 2 medium
    ones (about 360g/12¾oz)
    will make enough for 1 person,
    and scale up accordingly
vegetable oil (nope, not olive oil
    or sunflower – go old school!)

Sometimes you just need something plain, simple and satisfying when you're feeling down – and that's where our good friend Paul Hawkins comes in. He can sure make a mean roast potato. He holds this recipe as close to his chest as his heaving, lusty bosoms will allow, but, readers, he's letting you have it. Not because he owes me a favour or 'owt.

You might think it's a pretty basic thing to throw into this collection of fantastic recipes, but hear me out: is there a bigger joy in this world than biting into a perfect roast potato? One that is crunchy on the outside and fluffy and lovely on the inside? No. So shush – and get these made.

Peel the potatoes with all the care you'd show if you were defusing a bomb – these need to be perfect. Then cut them on the diagonal into decent-sized chunks. Put them into a pan of salted water so they're covered, and boil for 7 minutes.

Drain off the water, then pop the lid on and give the potatoes a good rough and tumble until they fluff up – if some break apart, it doesn't matter – more crispy bits later. Let them sit in the pan with the lid on for an hour. The 'steaming' part is essential: don't miss it out.

Preheat the oven to 200°C fan/425°F/gas mark 7. Take a shallow roasting pan and pour in about 1cm (½ inch) of vegetable oil. Pop it on the top shelf of the oven for 10 minutes, to heat up.

Working quickly and carefully, place the potatoes in the hot oil, giving each one space to breathe and coating them with the oil – add the bits of potato that fell off too, they'll be like potato crackling – then it's straight back into the oven for 20 minutes.

After 20 minutes, out comes the tin, turn and baste the potatoes, and back in.

Repeat after another 20 minutes. One more turn and baste, then leave them in for another 10 minutes.

After 10 minutes out they come, assuming they're golden and full of crispy edges. Sitting in the oil will simply soften them.

Try to enjoy your dinner through the film of rapturous tears in your eyes.

Notes from Paul (Hawkins)
- *You know when people say size isn't important – well, it bloody is here. Smaller uniform potatoes will lead to lots of crispy edges.*
- *You could serve these with a roast, but honestly, a bowlful of these with beans and cheese is absolute and utter comfort food.*

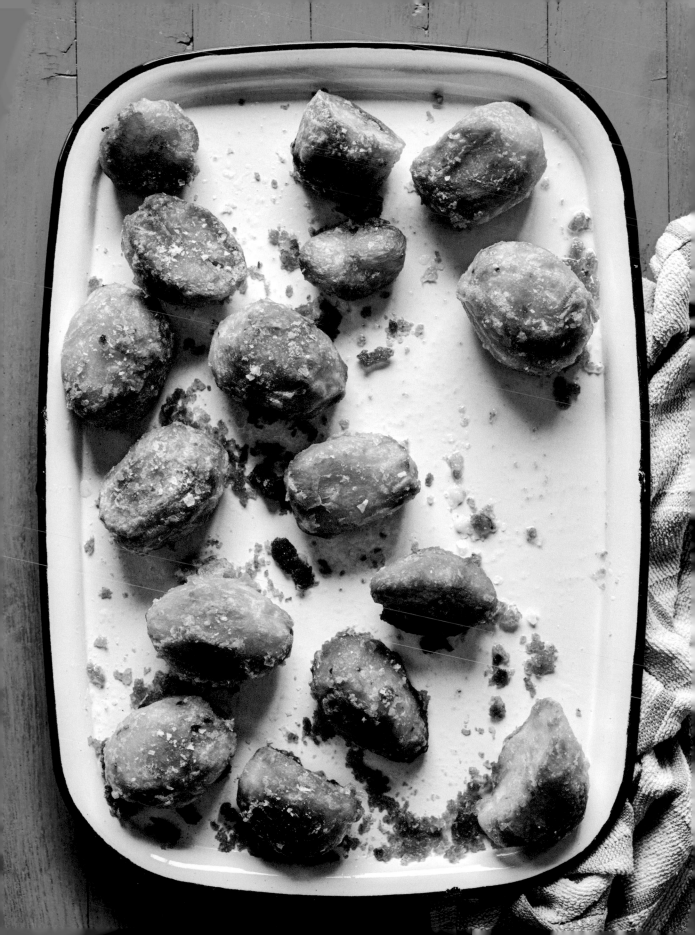

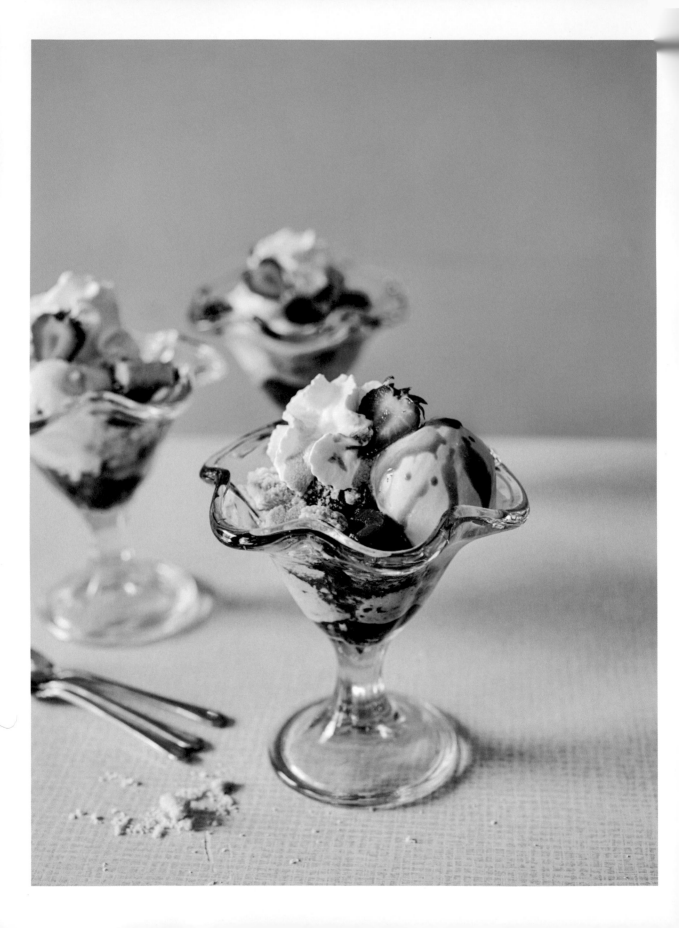

STRAWBERRY SHORTCAKE ICE CREAM SUNDAE

Serves 4
523 calories

You're looking at this and thinking you can't have such decadence on a diet. Listen, we understand, we used to think the same thing, but this is one of our cheat's recipes where a little of what you fancy does you good. When you've had a week of slimming meals and fancy a treat, this is something to savour and enjoy.

We tend to have something like this every couple of weeks to scratch the 'need sugar, can almost see my feet again' itch, and we very much encourage you to do the same. Life isn't there to be filled with fruit salads and rice cakes, after all.

However, this is still a diet book, so if you want to slim it down a little, there are plenty of replacements you can make which are listed in Paul's notes below. But sometimes – just sometimes – it's worth going the whole hog.

300g (10½oz/3 cups) strawberries, chopped, plus 4 strawberries, cut into halves
2 tablespoons sugar
250g (9oz) strawberry ice cream
12 shortbread fingers
250g (9oz) vanilla ice cream
whipped cream

Heat a saucepan over a medium-low heat and add the chopped strawberries along with the sugar. Simmer for 7–10 minutes, stirring occasionally, to make a strawberry sauce, then remove from the heat and allow to cool.

Take 4 sundae glasses or bowls and put a tablespoon of the strawberry sauce into the bottom of each one, followed by a scoop of strawberry ice cream.

Crumble over 2 shortbread fingers, and add a scoop of vanilla ice cream.

Spoon over some more of the strawberry sauce, followed by another 2 crumbled shortbread fingers.

Top each sundae with a swirl of whipped cream and 2 strawberry halves.

Notes from Paul

- *There's a whole raft of ice creams out there now that take pleasure in telling you how low in calories they are – they're really rather good and worth exploring, although if you're anything like us, you won't be able to have half a tub in the freezer without shooting the kitchen angst-ridden glances all night until you succumb.*
- *Shortbread fingers can be swapped out for ladyfingers – those wee sponge fingers that your gran used to put in her trifle – which sounds like an awful euphemism but I hand-on-heart promise it isn't.*
- *Strawberry jelly, made the night before and scattered with chopped strawberries before it sets, makes a perfectly acceptable substitute for the sticky strawberry sauce.*
- *You could always have an apple and a cry in the hallway cupboard if you were so inclined.*

RECIPE NOTES

BREAKFAST

NEAPOLITAN OVERNIGHT OATS

STORE/MAKE AHEAD: We have found overnight oats last perfectly fine for 3 days in the fridge as long as they're in a good sealed jar.

DARK CHOCOLATE & ORANGE BAKED OATS

FREEZE: The recipe can be doubled or tripled and baked in individual ramekins as per the recipe, then, once cool, wrapped individually in clingfilm and popped into a freezer bag. They'll keep for 1 month in the freezer. Defrost overnight, then unwrap and reheat in the microwave until piping hot.

STORE/MAKE AHEAD: You can make this the night before, chill overnight and warm up in a 180°C fan/400°F/gas mark 6 oven for 10 minutes in the morning (or microwave until piping hot, as long as they're in a microwave-safe dish).

TOAST TOPPERS

Stewed tomatoes with a chilli kick
STORE/MAKE AHEAD: This topping can be made ahead of time and kept chilled in a sealed container for up to 3 days. It can then be warmed in a pan over a gentle heat.

FULL ENGLISH BREAKFAST QUICHE

FREEZE: Slice when cold, then wrap each slice in foil and freeze. Grab a wedge the night before to defrost for breakfast.

STORE/MAKE AHEAD: Allow to cool, then cover and chill for up to 3 days. Can be eaten cold or warmed in a 180°C fan/400°F/gas mark 6 oven for 10–20 minutes until piping hot.

LUNCH & LIGHT BITES

GRANNY'S GARDEN FRITTATA

FREEZE: Allow to cool, then slice and wrap individually in clingfilm and pop into a sandwich bag. Allow to defrost overnight in the fridge before eating.

STORE/MAKE AHEAD: Allow to cool, then chill, covered, for up to 3 days. Eat cold or reheat in a 180°C fan/400°F/gas mark 6 oven for 10–20 minutes, or in a microwave on low power, until piping hot.

A RIGHT NICE MINESTRONE SOUP

STORE/MAKE AHEAD: To make ahead, prepare the soup as per the recipe but don't add the pasta to the soup. Chill the soup and cooked pasta separately in sealed containers for up to 2 days. When ready to eat, reheat the soup in a pot over a low heat and, once hot, stir through the cooked pasta.

SLOW COOKED CHEESY BROCCOLI SOUP

FREEZE: Prepare the soup as in the recipe, but don't sprinkle on the grated cheese. Allow the soup to cool, then pour into airtight containers and freeze for up to 2 months. Defrost overnight in the fridge (it may look a bit watery, which is fine).

Reheat over a low heat in a large pan. Serve sprinkled with the grated cheese.

STORE/MAKE AHEAD: Prepare the soup as in the recipe, but don't sprinkle on the grated cheese. Allow the soup to cool completely, then pour into airtight containers. Chill for up to 2 days.

Reheat over a low heat in a large pan. Serve sprinkled with the grated cheese.

CHOPPED COUSCOUS SALAD

STORE/MAKE AHEAD: Chill in an airtight container for up to 2 days.

CHEESY CHUBBY FISHCAKES

FREEZE: To freeze, lay the fried fishcakes on a baking sheet lined with baking paper. Freeze uncovered for 1–2 hours (or until solid), then transfer the fishcakes to a resealable bag and freeze for up to 3 months. Allow the fishcakes to defrost in the fridge overnight, then reheat on a baking sheet in a 180°C fan/400°F/gas mark 6 oven for 10–15 minutes, until piping hot.

STORE/MAKE AHEAD: To make ahead, assemble the fishcakes and coat with the breadcrumbs, but don't fry them. Place on a baking sheet and cover with clingfilm, then chill for up to 1 day. When ready to cook, uncover the fishcakes and fry as instructed in the recipe.

PROPER HAM AND EGG QUICHE

FREEZE: Allow to cool, then slice and wrap individually in clingfilm and pop into a sandwich bag. Allow to defrost overnight in the fridge before eating.

STORE/MAKE AHEAD: Allow to cool, then chill, covered, for up to 3 days. Eat cold or reheat in a 180°C fan/400°F/gas mark 6 oven for 10–20 minutes, or in a microwave on low power, until piping hot.

MEAT-FREE MARVELS

ROASTED RAINBOW CARBONARA

FREEZE: You can freeze the spare egg whites.

STORE/MAKE AHEAD: You can roast the vegetables in advance and chill them for up to 3 days in an airtight container.

TOMATO & CHICKPEA STEW

FREEZE: Prepare as in the recipe but don't stir in the baby spinach.

Allow to cool, then freeze in an airtight container for up to 2 months. Defrost overnight in the fridge.

When ready to serve, warm up in a large pan over a low heat until hot, adding water if needed to loosen. Stir through the baby spinach until wilted.

STORE/MAKE AHEAD: Prepare as in the recipe but don't stir in the baby spinach.

Allow to cool, then chill in an airtight container for up to 2 days.

When ready to serve, warm up in a large pan over a low heat until hot, adding water if needed to loosen. Stir through the baby spinach until wilted.

CREAMY GARLIC MUSHROOMS ON CHEESY FRIED POLENTA

STORE/MAKE AHEAD: You can cook the polenta ahead of time and chill, covered, for up to 2 days.

THREE BEAN COWBOY STEW

FREEZE: Allow to cool, then freeze in an airtight container for up to 2 months. Defrost overnight in the fridge.

When ready to serve, warm up in a large pan over a low heat, adding water if needed to loosen, until hot. Serve with cooked rice.

STORE/MAKE AHEAD: Like all chillis, the longer you leave this the better it tastes – keep some aside for a jacket potato topping the next day.

STUFFED SPINACH & RICOTTA CANNELLONI

STORE/MAKE AHEAD: Cool completely, then chill, covered, for up to 3 days. Reheat in a 180°C fan/400°F/gas mark 6 oven for 15–20 minutes, covering with foil if needed to stop it drying out, until piping hot.

VEGETARIAN MOUSSAKA

STORE/MAKE AHEAD: Cool completely, then chill, covered, for up to 3 days. Reheat in a 180°C fan/400°F/gas mark 6 oven for 15–20 minutes, covering with foil if needed to stop it drying out, until piping hot.

FETA POTATO CAKES

FREEZE: Freeze the fried potato cakes on a baking sheet lined with baking paper, uncovered, for 1–2 hours or until solid. Transfer to a resealable bag and freeze for up to 3 months. To reheat, place a few frozen potato cakes on a baking sheet and bake in a 180°C fan/400°F/gas mark 6 oven for 15-20 minutes until fully defrosted and piping hot.

STORE/MAKE AHEAD: To make ahead, prepare until just before the frying step. Place on a baking sheet and cover, then chill for up to 3 days. When ready to eat, fry as per the recipe instructions.

LIGHTER SPANAKOPITA

STORE/MAKE AHEAD: Cool completely, then chill, covered, for up to 3 days. Reheat in a 180°C fan/400°F/gas mark 6 oven for 15-20 minutes, covering with foil if needed to stop it drying out, until piping hot.

CURRY LOAF RELOADED

FREEZE: Cool completely, then wrap in foil and place in a resealable food bag. Freeze for up to 2 months. Defrost overnight in the fridge before eating.

STORE/MAKE AHEAD: Cool completely, then wrap in clingfilm. Chill for up to 2 days. Eat cold, or reheat leftovers in a microwave on low, or in an oven (covered with foil if needed to prevent it drying out) at 180°C fan/400°F/gas mark 6 for 10–15 minutes, until hot.

WEEKDAY DINNERS

HAM & PINEAPPLE PASTA BAKE

STORE/MAKE AHEAD: Allow to cool completely, then chill, covered, for up to 3 days. Reheat, covered with foil, in a 180°C fan/400°F/gas mark 6 oven for 15 to 20 minutes until piping hot.

LAMB & HALLOUMI MEATBALLS

FREEZE: These freeze perfectly: arrange them on a baking tray, put that into the freezer and, once they're frozen, pop them into a sandwich bag.

STORE/MAKE AHEAD: Allow to cool completely, then chill, covered, for up to 3 days. Reheat the meatballs in their sauce in a large pan over a low heat until piping hot – you may need to add a splash of water to thin the sauce as you do this.

PESTO LAMB STEAKS

STORE/MAKE AHEAD: The pesto can be made ahead and kept chilled in an airtight container for up to 3 days.

PROPER HEARTY BEEF & VEG SOUP

STORE/MAKE AHEAD: To make ahead, prepare the recipe until just before you add the cabbage. Allow to cool completely, then chill in an airtight container for up to 2 days. Reheat in a large pan over a low heat until simmering and allow to simmer for a further 20 minutes, adding water as needed to maintain the soupy texture. Add the cabbage and cook for a further 5 minutes.

FIVE-ALARM CHILLI

FREEZE: Allow to cool, then freeze in an airtight container for up to 2 months. Defrost overnight in the fridge.

When ready to serve, warm up in a large pan over a low heat, adding a splash of water if needed to loosen, until hot.

WEEKEND DINNERS

ULTIMATE COMFORT CHICKEN SOUP

FREEZE: Cool completely, then transfer to an airtight container and freeze for up to 2 months. Defrost overnight in the fridge. Reheat in a large pan over a low heat until gently simmering. Allow to simmer for 10 minutes before serving.

STORE/MAKE AHEAD: Cool completely, then transfer to an airtight container and chill for up to 3 days. Reheat in a large pan over a low heat until gently simmering. Allow to simmer for 10 minutes before serving.

OH THE HUMANITY CHICKEN

STORE/MAKE AHEAD: Cool any leftovers within 2 hours of cooking (removing the meat from the carcass and spreading it out on a baking sheet is a good way to do this), then chill in an airtight container for up to 2 days. Eat cold in sandwiches or reheat in a soup or stew.

SUPER TASTY TURKEY MEATBALLS

FREEZE: Freeze the shaped, uncooked meatballs on a baking sheet for 1–2 hours, until firm, then pop them into a resealable bag and freeze for up to 2 months. When ready to cook, allow the meatballs to defrost overnight in the fridge, then continue with the recipe as usual.

STORE/MAKE AHEAD: Allow to cool completely, then chill, covered, for up to 3 days. Reheat the meatballs in their sauce in a large pan over a low heat until piping hot; you may need to add a splash of water to thin the sauce as you do this.

GROATY PUDDING

STORE/MAKE AHEAD: Cool, then chill in an airtight container for up to 3 days. Reheat in a pan over a low heat, adding extra water as needed to loosen, until piping hot.

SPICY MEXICAN BEEF

STORE/MAKE AHEAD: To make ahead, cook until just before you add the runner beans. Allow the beef to cool completely, then chill for up to 3 days. Reheat in a large pot over a low heat until simmering, adding more water to loosen as needed. Add the runner beans, cook for 15 minutes, and serve.

FAKEAWAYS

FISH CURRY

FREEZE: You can freeze the aromatics (see ONE POT PHO) for up to 3 months. No need to defrost in advance, just tip into a hot pan with a few sprays of oil before continuing with the recipe.

STORE/MAKE AHEAD: You can prep the aromatics ahead of time by following the first step of the recipe (cooking the onion, garlic and ginger in the spices). This mixture can be kept in an airtight container in the fridge for up to 3 days.

CHICKEN TIKKA MASALA

FREEZE: Allow to cool completely, then freeze for up to 3 months. Defrost overnight in the fridge the day before you want to eat it. Reheat by warming in a large pan over a low heat, adding a splash of water if needed to loosen, until piping hot.

STORE/MAKE AHEAD:Allow to cool completely, then transfer to an airtight container and chill for up to 2 days. Reheat by warming in a large pan over a low heat, adding a splash of water if needed to loosen, until piping hot.

QUICK & EASY CHICKEN CURRY

FREEZE: Allow to cool, then freeze for up to 3 months. Allow to defrost overnight in the fridge the day before you want to eat it. Reheat by warming in a large pan over a low heat, adding a splash of water if needed to loosen, until piping hot.

STORE/MAKE AHEAD: Allow to cool completely, then chill in airtight containers for up to 2 days. Reheat by warming in a large pan over a low heat, adding a splash of water if needed to loosen, until piping hot.

ONE POT PHO

FREEZE: You can freeze the aromatic stock and chicken for up to 3 months (see below). Defrost overnight in the fridge before using. Reheat the stock and shredded chicken together in a large pan over a low heat, until piping hot, before continuing with the recipe as usual.

STORE/MAKE AHEAD: Prepare the aromatic stock and chicken ahead of time. Follow the recipe up until you pour the stock through a sieve. Allow the stock and shredded chicken to cool. Transfer the stock to an airtight container, and place the chicken in a resealable bag. Chill for up to 2 days. Reheat the stock and shredded chicken together in a large pan over a low heat, until piping hot, before continuing with the recipe as usual.

MONGOLIAN BEEF

STORE/MAKE AHEAD: Allow to cool completely, then transfer to an airtight container and chill for up to 2 days. Reheat in a non-stick pan, adding a splash of water to loosen if needed, set over a medium heat until piping hot.

A BIT ON THE SIDE

BACON & ROASTED SPROUTS WITH A CREAMY GARLIC SAUCE

STORE/MAKE AHEAD: To make ahead, follow the recipe until the step just before you mix everything together. Allow the sauce and roasted sprouts to cool completely. Chill in separate airtight containers for up to 3 days. When ready to eat, spread the roasted sprouts and pancetta on a baking tray and reheat in a 200°C fan/425°F/gas mark 7 oven for 10–15 minutes. Meanwhile, warm the cheese sauce in a pan over a low heat until piping hot. Toss the sprouts and sauce with the rocket and serve.

5 FAB SIMPLE SIDES:

Perfect coleslaw
STORE/MAKE AHEAD: Keep leftovers in an airtight container in the fridge for up to 3 days.

Bulgur wheat salad
STORE/MAKE AHEAD: Keep cooled leftovers in an airtight container in the fridge for up to 3 days. Eat cold or reheat in a frying pan, stirring over a medium heat until warmed through.

TREAT YOURSELF

CHERRY BAKEWELL CHEESECAKE SHOTS

STORE/MAKE AHEAD: These can be made the day before you want to serve them and kept covered in the fridge overnight.

TROPICAL PARFAIT

STORE/MAKE AHEAD: These can be made the day before you want to serve them and kept covered in the fridge overnight.

CHOCOLATE MOUSSE

STORE/MAKE AHEAD: These can be made the day before you want to serve them and kept covered in the fridge overnight.

BANANA & CUSTARD

STORE/MAKE AHEAD: Make the custard ahead of time, allow to cool, then keep in the fridge in an airtight container for up to 3 days. Reheat in a pan over a low heat until warmed through.

CHOCOLATE BANANA BREAD

STORE/MAKE AHEAD: Keep leftovers in an airtight container at room temperature for up to 5 days. If it gets a bit stale, toasting a slice will soften it.

THE OCCASIONAL BLOW OUT

THE BEST CHILLI MACARONI CHEESE

FREEZE: You can freeze the assembled macaroni cheese in its ovenproof dish before it has been baked. Allow to cool, then wrap in clingfilm followed by foil. Freeze for up to 3 months. Defrost overnight in the fridge, then unwrap and bake as instructed. You may need to bake it for a bit longer to ensure it is hot in the centre.

STORE/MAKE AHEAD: Store cooled leftovers, covered, in the fridge for up to 3 days. Reheat in a 180°C fan/400°F/ gas mark 6 oven, covered with foil to stop it drying out, for 15–20 minutes until piping hot.

BACON JAM BACON BURGER

STORE/MAKE AHEAD: Make the bacon jam ahead of time. Allow to cool and chill in an airtight container in the fridge for up to 3 days. Bring to room temperature (or warm in a small pan over a low heat) before serving.

INDEX

A BIG THANK YOU

Massive thanks goes to everyone at Hodder & Stoughton and Yellow Kite for smiling politely at us while we forgot our security passes, snaffled their biscuits and left a strong smell of damp in every meeting room we were pushed into. Whilst everyone was amazing, special thanks must go to Lauren Whelan for persistently ringing me back in June and never taking no for an answer; Natalie Bradley for never once sending shirty emails about deadlines (kidding, always gorgeous); Caitriona Horne for being endlessly wonderful and positive in the face of seeing us corpse in front of camera; Rebecca Mundy for encouraging us to be the best we could be and Dom Gribben and Bella Martin for listening to our ramblings for a good solid six hours.

Mani fanx to hour tyreless copi-editur, Annie Lee, who maid sure they're were no errars in our righting. Kerry Torrens sweated through our recipes to make sure they're nutritionally sound and tasty, and for that we owe her everything. Clare Skeats made our vision of a colourful, happy book come to life better than anything we could have ever thought. Liz and Max Haarala Hamilton took the fantastic photos and demurred politely when we asked for Vaseline on the lens. Frankie Unsworth took the time to style our food – we can't believe how good our food can look, and, on a side note, do buy her book, it's a really terrific read! Jen Kay was our brilliant art director and prop stylist, and conveyed exactly the style we wanted and for that we love her. Finally, Claudette Morris was our Production Manager, and although we've probably pushed her onto hard liquor with our lax approach to deadlines, we're ever so grateful.

Thanks to India, Hugo, Brody and Dan for making our slop look palatable; Fab for wading through the filth that is our Instagram account and, indeed, everyone else who took the time to make us believe we could do this. A personal shout-out to the folks in the finance department at Hodder who have paid for our trip to America.

Endless gratitude to our moderators Lisa-Clare Fairbairn, Jeanette Armour and Vicky McDermott, who ran our group effortlessly while we focussed on the book. No amount of kind words can make up for the crap they've had to wade through, and they've always been incredibly supportive while doing it. We love them dearly.

A relieved thank you to Jo, Victoria and Katy who managed to make us sound halfway decent on their always hilarious podcast, *The Secret World of Slimming Clubs*.

Thanks to Vanessa Walker for telling us about the 'dolly-whacker' – she knows what we mean. Along similar, filthy lines, gratitude for Claire 'Hells Belles' who informed us she can't answer Instagram messages because she's too busy 'ringing the Devil's doorbell'. Can't imagine.

JAMES:

Thanks to Chris, Christine and Deborah, who paid polite lip service to the detail of the book while trying to hide the joy that I might be able to put them in a decent care home when they're older.

Congratulations to Paul Hawkins (39), who has not only shown me how exactly a potato should be treated, but who has also, finally, managed to get his name in print without a footnote of 'and there were no survivors'. Further thanks go to who I assume is his grandad, Martin, for allowing me to hole up in their sparkling residence while I excitedly 'type up blog intros'.

Much love to my Work Wife Emma Lebovitch who provided endless, noisy enthusiasm once I had explained exactly what a book was, and to my Work Dad Shane Ackers, who was there for every wobble, whinge and 'what the f*** am I doing?' with his sage advice, Marlboro Lights and tiny little legs. Paul says thank you to Emma Wallace and Danielle Spencer-Jones for getting pissed with him and keeping him focussed.

Thank you to Paul for allowing me to stay at home to build the blog and the book while he endlessly toiled. His faults may be innumerate and his face only a 4/10, but there's no one else that I could hope to have adventures like we have together. Much love to my little Shittyarse.

PAUL:

Massive thanks also to my friends in the MHLT for always being so supportive of me, especially in the early days of all of this, and especially to Sandra, Kerry, Andy, Lorna, Lynn, Dave and Adam, who always took the time to listen to my crap and give encouragement.

My thanks most of all to James, my muffin, who I couldn't have done this without, and wouldn't want to. Thanks for being my furry hot water bottle. Now you can buy me that dog.

US:

Many thanks indeed to every last one of you who have bought our book, read our blog, sent us nonsense, sent us nudes (we won't tell your wife, even though she sends them too – barking up the wrong tree there love), given us feedback or have taken the time to let us know you're thinking of us. You have no idea how amazing this all is for us – and we thank you, without sarcasm or insincerity, from the very bottom of our cholesterol-soaked hearts.

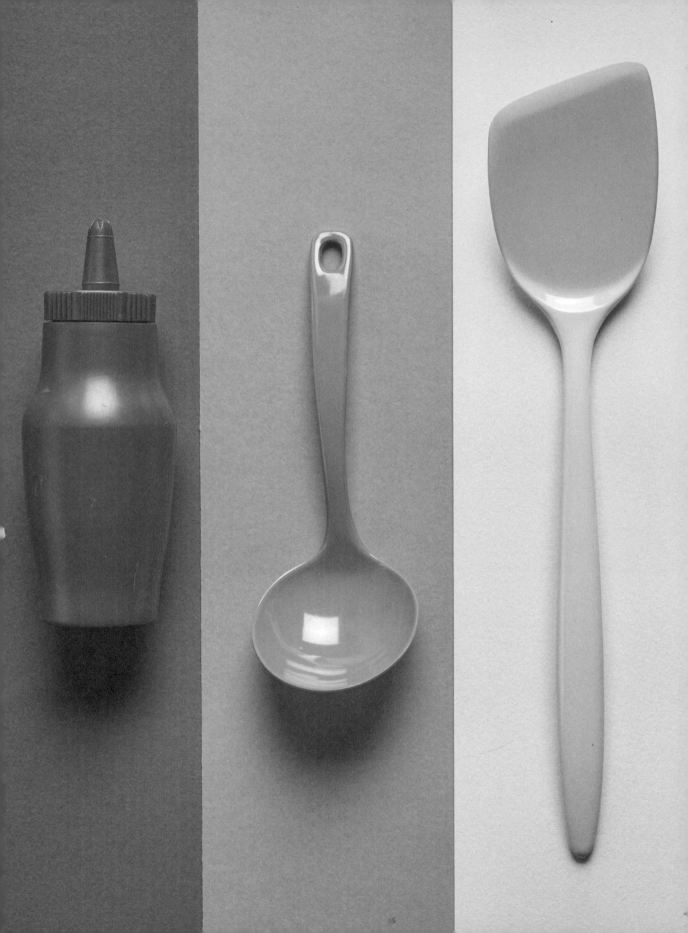